The Simplest Way to Lose Weight!

"From the thousands of letters I've received over the years from readers struggling with excess weight, I understand that no one wants to be bothered with counting calories or grams of carbs, fats, or protein...What you want is a straightforward, easy-to-follow, and effective plan for achieving and maintaining your ideal weight. And that's what my No Flour, No Sugar Diet is. How much more simple could a diet be than one that can be described in its entirety in just four words? No flour, no sugar. That's it. Simple, inexpensive, nutritious, and easy to maintain over the long haul."

—From DR. GOTT'S NO FLOUR, NO SUGAR DIET™

SUCCESS STORIES FOR
THIS REVOLUTIONARY PROGRAM
DR. GOTT'S NO FLOUR, NO SUGAR DIET™

"By following the No Flour, No Sugar Diet, I've lost 78 pounds in one year!"

—G.D., Skaneateles, NY

"I've tried every diet and diet pill known without any success. After four months on the No Flour, No Sugar Diet, I've already lost 45 pounds, and my quality of life is much improved."

—M.F., Salt Lake City, UT

...ase turn this page for more testimonials...

"My husband and I have been quite satisfied with what we consider to be our new way of living with food. My husband has lost 40 pounds and I have lost 25 to date, with more to come, I am certain."
—M.S., Naples, FL

"I am having good luck without sugar or flour in my diet. Most of all, I don't miss it. In 2 months I had lost 23 pounds, feel great, have more energy, and don't feel like I'm on a diet."
—B.C., Visalia, CA

"I've been on the No Flour, No Sugar Diet now about 2 months. It is great! I've lost 35 pounds and am still losing. It's very easy to follow. I feel much better, too."
—J.M., Lincoln, NE

"My husband and I lost 40 and 60 pounds respectively with the No Flour, No Sugar Diet. We also now walk 25 to 35 miles a week and are more active than ever."
—S.S., Auburn, IN

"I just love the No Flour, No Sugar Diet. I'm a cancer survivor of two years and my doctor is so pleased with my 25-pound weight loss and the fact that I'm feeling so good."
—B.H., Hanford, CA

"After I lost weight on Dr. Gott's No Flour, No Sugar Diet, I put on a pair of shorts for the first time and I realized the cellulite in my legs (which I've had since I was a teenager) was gone!"
—B.S., Whittier, CA

"I have lost 45 pounds on Dr. Gott's No Flour, No Sugar Diet. For me, the diet is easy."

—N.K., Groveton, TX

"I have never been overweight, but always had an extra 10 pounds that bothered me. Even with exercise and limiting calories, I could never keep them off permanently. It's only been 10 days, but I have effortlessly lost 3 pounds and the weight is steadily going down."

—J.G., Tallahassee, FL

"I've been following the No Flour, No Sugar Diet for about 18 months. I've lost 50 pounds, and it's been easy, too. Thanks."

—D.I., Anadarko, OK

"My husband lost 50 pounds and has kept it off. People who haven't seen him for a few months cannot believe how much weight he has lost. I am so proud of him."

—P.R., Stigler, OK

"I am 5'1" and weighed 234 pounds when I started Dr. Gott's No Flour, No Sugar Diet. I've been on it for four months and have lost 45 pounds."

—M.F. Princeton, NJ

"I have lost 80 pounds on the No Flour, No Sugar Diet."

—J.A., Columbia City, IN

"I've always had a problem with my weight and diets never worked for me. When I started Dr. Gott's No Flour, No Sugar Diet, I weighed 194 pounds. I am now at 146 pounds. I feel great!"

—V.G., Clovis, CA

Dr. Gott's
No Flour,
No Sugar
Diet™

Peter H. Gott, MD
with Robin Donovan

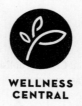

**WELLNESS
CENTRAL**

NEW YORK   BOSTON

Neither this diet nor any other diet should be followed without first consulting a health care professional. If you have any special conditions requiring attention, you should consult with your health care professional regularly regarding possible modification of the program contained in this book.

Wellness Central Edition

This Hachette Book Group USA edition is published by arrangement with Quill Driver Books/Word Dancer Press, Inc. 1254 Commerce Way, Sanger, CA 93657

Wellness Central
Hachette Book Group USA
237 Park Avenue
New York, NY 10017

Visit our Web site at www.HachetteBookGroupUSA.com.

Printed in the United States of America

Originally published in hardcover by Hachette Book Group USA.

First Wellness Central Trade Edition: May 2008
10 9 8 7 6 5 4 3 2 1

Wellness Central is an imprint of Grand Central Publishing.
The Wellness Central name and logo are trademarks of Hachette Book Group USA, Inc.

ISBN 978-0-446-17790-0 (pbk.)
LCCN: 2006937918

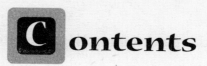ontents

Introduction...ix

— Part I —
The No Flour, No Sugar Basics

1 How and Why the No Flour, No Sugar Diet Works........4

2 Fueling Your Body for Optimal Health........................7

3 What's So Bad About Flour and Sugar?.....................13

4 Enough About What You Shouldn't Eat—

Let's Talk About What You Should Eat..............18

— Part II —
A New Lifestyle for a Better Life—
Tools to Help You Make Healthier Choices

5 Setting Realistic Goals...25

6 Write It Down: Keeping a Food Journal......................30

7 Reading the Fine Print: The Importance of Studying

Food Labels..34

8 Portion Control..39

9 Getting the Support You Need.....................................42

10 Don't Forget to Move: The Importance of Exercise......44

11 Planning for Success...50

12 The No Flour, No Sugar Diet

and Specific Medical Conditions.......................56

13 Busting Myths and Avoiding Negative "Remedies" 66

14 Staying on Track 76

15 Keep It Off: Maintaining Weight Loss Once You Have

      Reached Your Goal 81

— Part III —
Getting Down to Business: Your New Eating Plan

16 What to Eat/What not to Eat 86

17 Satisfying Your Sweet Tooth without Sugar 89

18 Satisfying Your Carbohydrate Cravings without Flour .. 96

19 The Meal Plans 99

— Part IV —
The Recipes

20 Breakfast 107

21 Soups, Salads, and Wraps 116

22 Snacks and Appetizers 133

23 Entrees 140

24 Side Dishes 167

25 Desserts 174

Index 179

About the Author 187

Introduction

Obesity is the second leading cause of preventable death in the U.S.—only smoking kills more people.

A few years ago, I got a letter from a reader who wrote, "What is the basis for the uproar about fat people? I think the issue is purely cosmetic. I'm proud of being overweight and I'm tired of being criticized for it. In my view, this is nothing more than discrimination."

In our society where "thin is in," there is certainly a good deal of discrimination against overweight people based on looks. While previous generations viewed stoutness as attractive, the pendulum has swung back and, as a culture, we now worship thinness—as evidenced by the constant bombardment of images of impossibly thin celebrities. But the problem is far from "purely cosmetic." There are serious recognized health consequences that stem from being overweight, including high blood pressure, elevated blood cholesterol, diabetes, cardiovascular disease, and many types of cancer.

The unfortunate truth is that Americans are fat, and getting fatter by the minute. Recent studies by the Centers for Disease Control reveal that 65 percent of American adults are overweight—up from 47 percent just twenty-five years ago. Worse, the rate of obesity has more than doubled in that time. In 1980, 15 percent of American adults were clinically obese. Today that number has ballooned to 31 percent.

According to the American Obesity Association, extremely overweight people have a greater than 70 percent chance of having an obesity-related health issue—including coronary artery disease, hypertension, diabetes, high blood cholesterol, and certain types of cancer. In fact, obesity is responsible for at least 300,000 deaths annually in the United States.

The seriousness of the health consequences of being overweight cannot be underestimated. And, adding insult to injury, obesity places enormous social and psychological stresses on individuals' lives in our thin-worshipping culture.

Any number of causes explain the stretching of our waistbands from coast to coast—from the supersizing of food portions to our decreasing intake of fresh fruits and vegetables and evermore sedentary lifestyles.

While there is some evidence that obesity has a genetic component and that heredity plays a role in a propensity for weight gain, our genes, on their own, can't explain the sharp rise in obesity rates over the past twenty-five years. Such a dramatic rise can only be explained by changes in our food choices and levels of physical activity.

Our parents may pass on to us genes that predict whether or not we will have a tendency to become overweight, but the lifestyle choices we learn from our families will likely have an even more profound effect on our weight and fitness level throughout life. From activity levels to eating patterns and food choices, we learn by example. If our parents and other family members regularly eat fried foods and rich desserts and rarely do more exercise than that involved in finding the remote control for the television, we're likely to grow up to have poor eating and exercise habits ourselves—and to be overweight adults.

Some people learn from their families to use food as a drug to cure feelings of sadness, loneliness, or anxiety. If you're one of those people, you may have developed a habit of overeating as a response to depression, stress at work or at home, boredom, or any number of difficult emotional issues. These patterns, too, are often passed down through generations.

Probably the worst culprit of all, though, is our ever-growing penchant for conserving energy while consuming ever larger portions of food. Rapidly proliferating fast food restaurants, convenience stores everywhere you look, and supermarkets bursting with high-fat, high-calorie ready-made meals combine with an automobile culture and omnipresent energy-saving devices to encourage us to consume more calories and to burn fewer.

The general consensus in the medical community is simple: We're eating too much of the wrong foods, too few of the right ones, and moving too little. The bottom line is that in order to lose weight, we need to eat fewer calories and exercise more.

"Experts" proclaiming they hold the secret to quick, easy, and lasting weight loss are a dime a dozen. Around every corner lurk devilish diet pushers, eager to sell you the Next Big Thing in weight loss: from diet pills and herbal supplements to low-fat, no-fat, low-carb, no-carb, high-protein, whole-grain, no-pain diets that promise to whisk your extra weight away with ease. Fad diets promise fast and dramatic results—and they often deliver on that promise. But on close examination, fad diets work not because they are high in one nutrient, low in another, or combine different nutrients in some magical combination; these diets cause weight loss for the simple reason that they are low in calories. Unfortunately, most fast-acting diets are detrimental to overall health, because they eliminate or severely restrict certain categories of important nutrients.

Low carbohydrate diets, the latest cure du jour, can, for instance, be potentially harmful because by focusing on limiting the intake of carbohydrates and increasing the intake of protein, they may encourage people to eat diets high in saturated fat and low in fiber-rich and vitamin-rich fruits and vegetables. This translates into an increased risk for heart disease, obesity, and (possibly) cancer. Furthermore, a very high protein diet stresses the kidneys and liver, forcing these organs to work harder to process and excrete the excess nitrogen proteins contain. The risk of osteoporosis, too, is accentuated because diets high in protein lead to calcium excretion. To make matters worse, these diets tend to be low in cholesterol-lowering fiber.

Dear Dr. Gott, *Over my lifetime, I have tried several diets (e.g., grapefruit, liquid diet, low-fat, Weight Watchers, etc.) with varying degrees of success. However, I always felt deprived and "on a diet," which made it difficult to follow over a period of time, and I ultimately gained back a good portion of the weight I had lost. Although never greatly overweight, I always found that to lose the last fifteen to twenty pounds was never easy. (I like to eat!) I couldn't keep it off. Well, for Lent, I decided to give up sugar and flour and follow the diet you have written about several times.*

What results! Over a four-week period, I have lost ten pounds and, amazingly enough, do not feel as though I am on a diet!

Do I miss bread, pasta, and desserts? Yes, but I do not consider myself deprived. I was even on a trip to Europe where I did not have their fine breads and sweets, but I didn't watch my intake of other items, either. I came home and found I had amazingly lost three more pounds.

I found the diet simple as well as easy to follow and (where it counts most) it has enabled me to lose weight.

While success stories abound about people who have lost weight on fad diets, almost all of those people gain the weight back—and often even more—as soon as they return to normal eating habits. These regimens are so restrictive that dieters cannot stick with them. Therefore, while they initially shed unwanted pounds, eventually they return to their previous eating patterns. Because they lost weight by practicing a rigorously restrictive diet, rather than by learning effective and healthful techniques for maintaining their ideal weight, they quickly gain back the unwanted pounds. Studies have documented that more than 90 percent of fast weight-losers eventually gain back most, if not all, of the weight they lost.

Weight loss achieved by severely restrictive diets has been shown, time and again, to be nearly impossible to sustain over time. Serial dieters, then, find themselves stuck in a perpetual loss-gain cycle that can lead to serious health problems, including elevated blood cholesterol levels and heart disease.

My No Flour, No Sugar program is more than a diet. It's a sensible guide for healthful eating that will help you achieve your goal weight and maintain it—and your overall well being—throughout your life. From the thousands of letters I've received over the years from readers struggling with excess weight, I understand that no one wants to be bothered with counting calories or grams of carbs, fats, or protein. You don't want to memorize daunting lists of foods that are allowable versus those that are not, or struggle with complicated formulas for combining foods from different food groups. And you don't want to be stuck eating nothing but grapefruit, cabbage soup, or even bacon.

What you want is a straightforward, easy to follow, and effective plan for achieving and maintaining your ideal weight. And that's what my No Flour, No Sugar Diet is. How much more simple could a diet be than one that can be described in its entirety in just four words? No flour, no sugar. That's it. Simple, inexpensive, easy to follow, nutritious, and easy to maintain over the long haul. There are no complicated instructions, no lists to memorize, and nothing to count or calculate. All you need to do is eliminate flour and added sugar from your diet. That means no bread, bagels, cookies, or cakes, but it doesn't mean you can't still enjoy lean meats, rice, low-fat dairy products, vegetables, and fruits.

Some people have taken me to task for allowing the use of artificial sweeteners in my diet since, regardless of their being FDA-approved, there are some concerns about their safety. My theory is that many of the people who need to lose weight are not going to be successful without using sugar substitutes. Being obese, or even moderately overweight, is an undebatable, serious health risk that takes precedence over the possible dangers of reasonable use of artificial sweeteners. Lose the weight first, then cut out artificial sweeteners if you can.

At last count, more than 260,000 people have requested information on my No Flour, No Sugar Diet and have had, as far as I know, success with it. Now I am pleased to find that the ease, simplicity, and effectiveness of the diet has made this book a *New York Times* bestseller, meaning thousands more are losing weight every day.

You'll find the diet so simple to follow and to integrate into your lifestyle that sticking to it will be a breeze compared to many of the more complicated or restrictive diets that have come and gone from the headlines over the years. And best of all, the diet is flexible enough to suit a variety of needs and weight-loss goals. For instance, once you've achieved your desired weight, you can begin to reintroduce flour-based foods such as pasta and bread into your diet while continuing to avoid sweets. If you begin to regain the weight, simply go back to following the more restrictive plan until the weight comes off again. Because the diet allows you to eat foods from all the food groups, you'll be able to get all the nutrients you need to maintain a healthy body while still reducing your caloric intake enough to lose extra pounds.

I developed my No Flour, No Sugar Diet over my nearly 40 years of medical practice to provide my patients with a simple method for losing weight that does not require spending large amounts of money, having to weigh portions or calculate calories, or enduring the nuisance associated with highly restrictive diet plans. I have received letters from thousands of readers who have lost phenomenal amounts of weight on my diet and have been able to maintain the losses easily by monitoring their weight and fine-tuning the diet to deal with the normal ups and downs of weight experienced in day-to-day life.

Your commitment to weight control is really a commitment to behavior control. You are more likely to succeed if you focus on changing your eating and activity patterns, not simply on losing pounds. Your goals need to be flexible, realistic, and implemented slowly. Changing lifelong behavior patterns can't be done overnight. Remember, it probably took many years for you to gain all those unwanted pounds; it's likely to take some time to shed them. Be prepared for plateaus and setbacks. After all, nobody's perfect so it's unrealistic to expect perfection of yourself. You are, however, capable of gradually developing the new behaviors and self-control skills that will make you a permanent winner in the battle of the bulge. Every day I get letters from readers who have had great success with my No Flour, No Sugar Diet. I hope you'll make the decision now to join them.

Part I

The No Flour, No Sugar Basics

Dear Dr. Gott, You should get some type of award for your No Flour, No Sugar Diet. I tried it and found that it is easy, cheap, and effective. I lost six pounds the first week, four pounds the second, and two pounds a week over the past three months. Thank you. Thank you.

In the forty years that I have practiced medicine, I have been impressed by the number of overweight people who yearn for a simple and inexpensive diet that they can feel comfortable following for extended periods. That is why I devised my No Flour, No Sugar Diet. That's it in a nutshell. If you want to lose weight steadily and consistently, limit your food intake to modest portions of meat, fish, poultry, whole grains, vegetables, salads, and fresh fruit. Avoid products that contain flour and added sugar and you'll easily cut enough calories from your diet to lose weight at the one or two pounds a week rate that is recommended by most medical experts.

Understanding just how the diet works, as well as a little bit about how your body utilizes the energy and nutrients provided by the foods you eat, will help you incorporate the diet into your life and shed excess pounds—and teach you how to make good food choices that will keep you active and fit for the rest of your life.

How and Why the No Flour,
No Sugar Diet Works

My No Flour, No Sugar Diet is not a magic pill, rather, it is a sensible way of eating that you'll find easy to adopt, inexpensive to practice, and simple to maintain for the rest of your life. You'll lose weight the optimal way—slowly but surely—and you'll feel great, too. As I mentioned, fad diets require you to make drastic changes in your diet for rapid, if unhealthful, weight loss. My No Flour, No Sugar Diet involves incremental changes that will have long-term beneficial effects on your weight and your overall health.

No flour, no sugar = fewer calories

The key to weight loss is simply to burn more calories than you take in. In the simplest of terms, then, my No Flour, No Sugar Diet works because eliminating flour and added sugar from your diet, without making other changes, reduces the number of calories you consume. I have found, and my patients' successes have verified, that eliminating flour and sugar from your diet is a simple way to cut calories instantly. Replacing high-calorie breads, for instance, with low-calorie vegetables and legumes will take a big chunk out of your caloric intake without leaving you feeling hungry or unsatisfied. Likewise, by replacing sugar and honey with no-calorie sweeteners, you can feed your sweet tooth while cutting calories.

To see how eliminating flour and sugar from your diet can dramatically reduce the number of calories you consume, let's compare the caloric content of two breakfasts—one with flour and sugar and one without. If you normally start your day with a bagel (about 250 calories) spread with a pat of butter (50 calories) and a tablespoon of strawberry jam (50 calories), and coffee with two teaspoons of sugar (30 calories), you're eating about 380 calories. Simply switching to old-fashioned oatmeal (100 calories) with one cup of skim milk (90 calories), a medium apple (80 calories), and coffee with artificial sweetener (0 calories), will save you 110 calories. You will also have reduced your fat intake from 7.5 grams to 2 grams, increased your fiber from 1 gram to 7 grams, and added 400 milligrams of calcium. And that's just breakfast.

As the above comparison clearly shows, eliminating flour and sugar from your diet is a simple way to rid your meals of many unnecessary calories. As an added bonus, you may find you'll automatically reduce the amount of fat you eat. Without bread and jelly, for instance, what fun is high-fat peanut butter? No flour means no cheesy pizza, no pasta in cream sauce, and no buttery cookies. Eliminating sugar means no more fat-laden ice cream or cake with buttercream frosting.

One pound of fat is equivalent to 3,500 calories. In order to lose one pound in a week, you need to consume 500 fewer calories a day or burn 500 more a day—or in a perfect world, a little of each. If you could make dietary changes such as those mentioned in the breakfast example above, cutting 110 calories from every meal you eat, you'd easily be more than half way there.

Avoid products containing any kind of flour, including wheat, rice, and corn flours, or refined or concentrated sugars (cane sugar, beet sugar, glucose, sucrose, high fructose corn syrup, maple syrup, honey, molasses, etc.). Whole grains and starchy vegetables, such as wheat berries, barley, brown rice, corn, and potatoes can add bulk to your meals. Satisfy your sweet tooth with fruit and products sweetened with fruit—as long as they don't contain added sugar. You can also enjoy sugar-free soda, chewing gum, and even many of the light ice creams now available that are sweetened with Splenda or other artificial sweeteners. Snack on raw vegetables and fresh fruit—excellent low-calorie sources of important nutrients and fiber.

Cutting the unnecessary, or "empty," calories of flour-based, sugary foods from your diet is a simple and relatively painless way to move toward your goal. Add an extra half hour of physical activity a day—a brisk walk, a game of tennis, or a spin on the treadmill—and you can expect easily to lose a pound a week until you reach your desired weight.

Slow and steady wins the race

While calorie reduction is the key to losing weight, it is important to remember that calories are our bodies' fuel. They provide the energy we need to perform normal daily activities. While consuming more calories than our bodies require leads to weight gain, it is important—even while you're trying to shed unwanted pounds—to eat enough calories to get the nutrients and energy your body requires to function optimally. That is why diet and health experts generally agree that the most effective diets are those on which you lose no more than one to two pounds per week.

To facilitate fast and dramatic weight loss, many fad diets require you to decrease your caloric intake to levels that are inadequate to insure you're getting the nutrients you need. Furthermore, weight that is lost quickly is very likely to come back just as fast when you stop starving your body. A slow, steady approach will maintain your health while producing the results you desire—and you're more likely to keep the weight off over time. You'll have a bad week here and there, but don't be discouraged. It happens to the best of us. Even if you don't meet your one-pound goal in a given week, stick with the diet and the weight loss will average out over time.

A diet for (just about) everyone

Because my No Flour, No Sugar Diet encourages eating a wide variety of foods from all of the food groups—including ample amounts of nutrient-rich fruits, vegetables, and whole grains—it is suitable for just about anyone, no matter what his or her age or activity level. Everyone, from young children to older adults, can benefit from cutting empty calories from highly processed foods out of their diet. People with specific medical conditions—including diabetes, coronary heart disease, high cholesterol, hypertension, and so on—are advised to seek the advice of the medical specialist who is treating them for that condition before making any major changes in their diet or activity level. That said, the No Flour, No Sugar Diet provides guidelines for healthy eating that can be adapted to suit a wide range of special dietary or medical needs.

The average American today consumes 500 more calories per day than in 1970.

Fueling Your Body for Optimal Health

With all the attention given to fad diets and different "expert'" opinions about what you should and shouldn't eat, it's easy to lose sight of what it means to eat a healthful diet.

As I discussed in the previous chapter, your body needs fuel to operate, and it gets this fuel from the food you eat. The amount of fuel you need is measured in calories and is based on your gender and age, as well as your daily activity level. You can calculate the number of calories you need by multiplying your current weight in pounds by 13 (15 if you are physically active). This calculation will give you an estimate of the number of calories you need to maintain your current weight. To lose weight at the recommended rate of one to two pounds per week, reduce your caloric intake by 500 calories per day.

The chart on the next page shows recommended calorie requirements by gender, age, and activity level.

The average American adult should consume somewhere between 2,000 and 3,000 calories per day—depending on age, gender, and activity level—to maintain his or her current weight. Unfortunately many of us consume far more calories than we burn because we fill up on junk food and sugary products, don't exercise, and make no effort to be prudent. Extra calories—those that are not metabolized for energy and health maintenance—are stored as fat. It is these extra calories that you should aim to eliminate as you strive to reach your optimal weight.

A balanced diet for a healthy body

Eating a healthful balance of nutritious foods and keeping total calorie consumption within the suggested range for your age, gender, and activity level are the keys not just to achieving your goal weight, but also to living a long and healthy life. Fad diets tend to focus on what you

Recommended Calorie Requirements

The chart below identifies the calorie levels for males and females by age and activity level. Calorie levels are provided for each year of childhood, from 2–18 years, and for adults in 5-year increments.

	MALES				FEMALES		
Activity level	Sedentary*	Mod. active*	Active*	Activity level	Sedentary*	Mod. active*	Active*
AGE				AGE			
2	1000	1000	1000	2	1000	1000	1000
3	1000	1400	1400	3	1000	1200	1400
4	1200	1400	1600	4	1200	1400	1400
5	1200	1400	1600	5	1200	1400	1600
6	1400	1600	1800	6	1200	1400	1600
7	1400	1600	1800	7	1200	1600	1800
8	1400	1600	2000	8	1400	1600	1800
9	1600	1800	2000	9	1400	1600	1800
10	1600	1800	2200	10	1400	1800	2000
11	1800	2000	2200	11	1600	1800	2000
12	1800	2200	2400	12	1600	2000	2200
13	2000	2200	2600	13	1600	2000	2200
14	2000	2400	2800	14	1800	2000	2400
15	2200	2600	3000	15	1800	2000	2400
16	2400	2800	3200	16	1800	2000	2400
17	2400	2800	3200	17	1800	2000	2400
18	2400	2800	3200	18	1800	2000	2400
19-20	2600	2800	3000	19-20	2000	2200	2400
21-25	2400	2800	3000	21-25	2000	2200	2400
26-30	2400	2600	3000	26-30	1800	2000	2400
31-35	2400	2600	3000	31-35	1800	2000	2200
36-40	2400	2600	2800	36-40	1800	2000	2200
41-45	2200	2600	2800	41-45	1800	2000	2200
46-50	2200	2400	2800	46-50	1800	2000	2200
51-55	2200	2400	2800	51-55	1600	1800	2200
56-60	2200	2400	2600	56-60	1600	1800	2200
61-65	2000	2400	2600	61-65	1600	1800	2000
66-70	2000	2200	2600	66-70	1600	1800	2000
71-75	2000	2200	2600	71-75	1600	1800	2000
76 and up	2000	2200	2400	76 and up	1600	1800	2000

* Calorie levels are based on the Estimated Energy Requirements (EER) and activity levels from the Institute of Medicine Dietary Reference Intakes Macronutrients Report, 2002.

Sedentary = less than 30 minutes a day of moderate physical activity in addition to daily activities.

Mod. Active = at least 30 minutes up to 60 minutes a day of moderate physical activity in addition to daily activities.

Active = 60 or more minutes a day of moderate physical activity in addition to daily activities.

(Source: USDA, www.MyPyramid.gov)

shouldn't eat, but it's important to remember that the foods you eat provide your body with all the nutrients it needs to perform daily bodily functions, maintain your organs, and allow you to live an active and fulfilling life.

In 2005, the United States Department of Agriculture (USDA) published its latest dietary guidelines, which emphasize maintaining healthful weight, stronger muscles and bones, and balanced nutrition to help prevent chronic illnesses such as heart disease, diabetes, and certain cancers. These new guidelines are reflected in an updated food guide pyramid, now known as "MyPyramid," which encourages you to increase your intake of fruits, vegetables, whole grains, and low-fat or nonfat milk and milk products while limiting consumption of saturated and trans fats, cholesterol, added sugars, salt, and alcohol. The guidelines are designed to encourage you to keep your body weight within healthful limits, to engage in regular physical activity, and to make smart food choices so that you get the most nutrition possible out of the calories you consume. More information on the new dietary guidelines and MyPyramid, including interactive tools, can be found at www.MyPyramid.gov. (See page 10.)

The most important message of the new dietary guidelines is that, while many fad diets encourage you to eliminate all foods from one food group or another, each of the food groups provides your body with important nutrients that, combined, keep you fit and healthy. Therefore, to maintain optimal health, you should eat foods from all three of the primary food groups—or "macronutrients," which include carbohydrates, fats, and proteins—as each has its own important function.

Carbohydrates

Carbohydrates may have gotten a bad rap lately, but they make up an extremely important food group—the one that provides most of the energy your body needs to perform its daily activities. Carbohydrates come from grains (wheat, rice, barley, oats, etc.), legumes, fruits, vegetables, and dairy products. As discussed later, the majority of your carbohydrate calories should come from minimally processed foods: whole grains, beans, fresh fruits, and vegetables.

Fats

Fats serve as stored energy that your body can draw on when not enough carbohydrates are available. They also provide fatty acids, which are crucial for the growth of body tissue, and enable your body to circulate, store, and

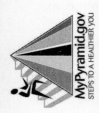

MyPyramid.gov
STEPS TO A HEALTHIER YOU

GRAINS Make half your grains whole	VEGETABLES Vary your veggies	FRUITS Focus on fruits	MILK Get your calcium-rich foods	MEAT & BEANS Go lean with protein
Eat at least 3 oz. of whole-grain cereals, breads, crackers, rice, or pasta every day	Eat more dark-green veggies like broccoli, spinach, and other dark leafy greens	Eat a variety of fruit	Go low-fat or fat-free when you choose milk, yogurt, and other milk products	Choose low-fat or lean meats and poultry
		Choose fresh, frozen, canned, or dried fruit		Bake it, broil it, or grill it
1 oz. is about 1 slice of bread, about 1 cup of breakfast cereal, or ½ cup of cooked rice, cereal, or pasta	Eat more orange vegetables like carrots and sweetpotatoes	Go easy on fruit juices	If you don't or can't consume milk, choose lactose-free products or other calcium sources such as fortified foods and beverages	Vary your protein routine — choose more fish, beans, peas, nuts, and seeds
	Eat more dry beans and peas like pinto beans, kidney beans, and lentils			

For a 2,000-calorie diet, you need the amounts below from each food group. To find the amounts that are right for you, go to MyPyramid.gov.

Eat 6 oz. every day	Eat 2½ cups every day	Eat 2 cups every day	Get 3 cups every day; for kids aged 2 to 8, it's 2	Eat 5½ oz. every day

Find your balance between food and physical activity

- Be sure to stay within your daily calorie needs.
- Be physically active for at least 30 minutes most days of the week.
- About 60 minutes a day of physical activity may be needed to prevent weight gain.
- For sustaining weight loss, at least 60 to 90 minutes a day of physical activity may be required.
- Children and teenagers should be physically active for 60 minutes every day, or most days.

Know the limits on fats, sugars, and salt (sodium)

- Make most of your fat sources from fish, nuts, and vegetable oils.
- Limit solid fats like butter, stick margarine, shortening, and lard, as well as foods that contain these.
- Check the Nutrition Facts label to keep saturated fats, *trans* fats, and sodium low.
- Choose food and beverages low in added sugars. Added sugars contribute calories with few, if any, nutrients.

absorb the important fat-soluble vitamins A, D, E, and K. Perhaps most important, fats make your food more enjoyable by adding flavor.

Saturated fats come mostly from animal sources (meat and dairy products), while unsaturated fats—both monounsaturated and polyunsaturated—come primarily from foods of plant origin and some seafood. A third type of fat, called trans fat, comes from vegetable oil that has been treated with hydrogen to make it more solid and longer lasting. You can recognize this type of fat on food labels because it is referred to as "hydrogenated" or "partially hydrogenated" oil.

While some fat is necessary for a healthy body, eating foods high in saturated or trans fats can lead to elevated blood cholesterol levels and an increased risk of heart disease and certain types of cancer. Both saturated and trans fats tend to raise LDL (the "bad" cholesterol) levels in the blood. Trans fat delivers a double whammy in that it also tends to lower HDL (the "good" cholesterol) levels as well.

Unsaturated fats in the diet do not lead to high blood cholesterol levels. Some studies have shown that eating foods that contain these fats can actually be beneficial by reducing the level of LDL cholesterol in the blood. Polyunsaturated fats, such as those found in safflower and corn oils, have been shown to lower both HDL and LDL, while foods containing monounsaturated fats, including olive and canola oils, avocados, and nuts, tend to lower only the bad cholesterol without affecting levels of good cholesterol.

Recent studies of the traditional diet of people who live in the region of the Mediterranean, a diet consisting primarily of fruits, vegetables, nuts, whole grains, and olive oil and emphasizing more "healthy fats" and fewer simple carbohydrates—have shown that consuming more monounsaturated fats, along with ample amounts of the phytochemicals, antioxidants, and fiber found in fresh fruits and vegetables, may lower the risk of obesity, high cholesterol, high blood pressure, and insulin resistance while protecting against cardiovascular risks. As a result, some physicians now counsel their patients to consume a Mediterranean-style diet that is rich in fruits, vegetables, whole grains, and unsaturated fats. Just what I've been preaching for years.

Proteins

Proteins are necessary for building and maintaining healthy body tissue, from internal organs to bones, muscles, and skin. Proteins come mostly from meat, poultry, seafood, dairy products, beans, nuts, and seeds. In order to limit the amount of saturated fat in your diet, it is best to opt for lean meats, poultry, seafood, low-fat or nonfat dairy products, and beans for your protein allotment.

Vitamins and minerals

While not one of the categories of macronutrients that supply your body with calories, vitamins and minerals are an important part of a healthful diet. They are like the lubrication in the gears of your body helping it to function optimally and ward off disease. Different vitamins and minerals can be found in grains, meat, fish, poultry, dairy products, vegetables, fruits, nuts, seeds, and legumes. Eating a wide variety of foods from different food groups ensures that you get all of the vitamins and minerals your body needs.

Dear Dr. Gott, My husband and I are too heavy and have begun your No Flour, No Sugar Diet with initial great success. However, our friends claim we won't lose weight if we eat fruit, unsweetened juice, potatoes, rice, carrots, corn, and peas. Are we on the right track?

Dear Reader, You seem to be. I believe that your friends ought to keep their opinions to themselves. Once you and your husband have lost substantial weight—which you should on my diet—they can eat crow, known for its low-calorie protein (just kidding). All vegetables, fruits, and meats are allowed on my diet—in moderation—and will help to make dieting less demanding. Remember to keep my diet simple: no flour, no sugar. That's it.

Choose "nutrient-dense" foods

Unfortunately, poor food choices lead many of us regularly to consume more calories than our bodies require without getting the nutrients we need. By choosing foods that are high in nutrients while still being low or moderate in calorie content, you can achieve and maintain your goal weight without feeling hungry or deprived and still remain healthy. The key is to opt for "nutrient-dense" foods. These include fruits, vegetables, legumes, whole grains, and lean meats that pack a high nutrition-to-calorie ratio.

3

What's So Bad About Flour and Sugar?

Flour and sugar are both carbohydrates, so what's so bad about them? It's not that these foods are bad because they are carbohydrates, but rather because added sugars and refined flour provide "empty calories," unlike their nutrient-dense cousins—whole grains, fruits, vegetables, and legumes—that provide fiber, vitamins, and minerals along with their carbohydrate punch.

The skinny on carbohydrates

Carbohydrates, as I've said before, are where your body gets most of the fuel it needs for everything from walking, talking, and dancing to thinking, pumping blood, and digestion. But in order to access that fuel, your body needs to break the carbohydrates down and convert them to the simple sugar known as glucose. Through digestion, your body breaks down the carbohydrates you consume—whether from whole grains, legumes, vegetables, or cake and candy bars—into glucose.

But all carbohydrates are not created equal. Simple carbohydrates such as cane sugar, beet sugar, corn syrup, honey, and maple syrup are made up of small sugar molecules or "simple sugars." This type of carbohydrate provides ready energy because your body has to do very little work to convert simple sugars to glucose. They are digested quickly and easily, sending a rush of glucose into your blood stream shortly after the food is consumed. When your blood is flooded with glucose in this way, you experience a temporary sugar "high" caused by the spike in your blood sugar level. A short time later, as the glucose leaves your system just as quickly as it entered it, you experience a "crash," which leaves you feeling fatigued and listless—and hungry again as your body craves more fuel.

To the contrary, "complex carbohydrates," such as whole grains (rice, wheat, oats, barley, quinoa, and corn), legumes, and vegetables are made up of much more complicated sugar molecules. Your body needs to work much harder to break these complex sugars down and convert them to glucose. Because of the extra effort required to digest these foods, digestion takes place over an extended period of time, and the glucose your body gets from these foods is released into your blood stream at a slower, steadier pace.

Just to confuse you further, the carbohydrates that come from fruits and milk products are considered simple carbohydrates. But because fruits and milk products are relatively low in sugar and provide big doses of important vitamins and minerals—fruits also provide fiber—these foods can be enjoyed as a regular part of a healthful diet. To make sure you are getting the biggest bang for your calories, opt for whole fresh fruits instead of sugary fruit juices, and choose low-fat or nonfat milk products.

Most experts recommend that 50 to 60 percent of the calories you eat come from carbohydrates. And most of these should be the complex type, which are digested slowly.

The bottom line is that the faster your body digests your food, the sooner you will be hungry again and the more you will eat in the long run. Foods that require more work to be digested will leave you feeling full for longer, and are less likely to lead you to overeat.

In addition to thinking about "good" carbohydrates versus "bad" carbohydrates based on how quickly they are digested, consider how much nutrition they provide. Most simple carbohydrates (cakes, cookies, candies) are made up of simple sugars and not much else. In contrast, complex carbohydrate foods such as whole grains, vegetables, and legumes—as well as nutrient-rich fresh fruits and low-fat and nonfat milk products—provide a host of essential nutrients, including vitamins, minerals, proteins, and healthful fats.

Fiber—calorie-free and good for you, too

Fiber is an important factor in determining how quickly your body digests carbohydrates. Fiber is a substance found in plant cell walls that cannot be digested by the human body, but it serves numerous important purposes nonetheless. Fiber has no calories—it is not broken down like other foods, but rather moves through your digestive system virtually intact—so it provides calorie-free filler, giving you a feeling of fullness from fewer calories when you consume foods that are high in fiber. Certain types of fiber also absorb water in the body, making you feel even more full.

Fiber has been shown to slow the digestive process, thus reducing the absorption of glucose, which, as we learned earlier, means you won't experience sharp increases and declines in your blood sugar levels. Eating high fiber foods, then, will help to regulate your blood sugar so that you don't experience those sugar crashes that leave you tired and hungry—and more likely to overeat.

As an added bonus, fiber also offers a host of other health benefits. It has been shown to help decrease blood cholesterol levels and the risk of certain types of cancer.

Fiber is found in whole grains (oats, wheat, brown rice, barley, etc.), as well as vegetables, fruits, and legumes.

Good grains gone bad

In 1970, the average American consumed about 116 pounds of wheat flour. By 2002, that figure had risen to more than 136 pounds a year. [From the U.S. Census Bureau's Statistical Abstract of the United States, 2002—http://www.census. gov/statab/www/]

While many a low-carb diet guru would have you believe that all carbohydrates are created equal—and are equally to blame for making you fat—they are just plain wrong. As I've said, fresh fruits and vegetables, as well as whole grains, are full of the essential vitamins, minerals, and fiber that we need to have healthy bodies, protect ourselves against disease, and function properly.

The problem arises when technology takes over the digestion process, removing all those valuable nutrients before we even have a chance to taste them, let alone put them to work.

Simply put, the more refined a carbohydrate is, the fewer nutrients it contains because it has already been broken down, by the refining process, to its elemental form. Modern processing technology has managed to take once healthful whole grains and strip them of their very benefits. The wheat grain, for instance, a veritable nutrition workhorse in its natural form, is steamed, pounded, and scraped to remove its outer fiber-full bran layer, its mineral-dense germ, and its vitamin-rich oil. Next it is pulverized by high-speed steel rollers into a fine powder, then bleached to remove any possible likeness to its original form. This powdery white substance is then labeled "all-purpose flour" and used to make almost all of the breads, cookies, crackers, cereals, and pastas you find on your supermarket shelves. Even those toasty brown "wheat breads" are often made with white flour and then artificially colored to make them look "healthy."

After all that processing, flour retains its high calorie nature but little else. It is virtually devoid of fiber and the vitamins and minerals our bodies need to function properly and fend off disease. The calories in all-purpose flour are what nutritionists call "empty calories." They will fill you up and provide instant energy, but they won't nourish your body for the long haul.

> **Dear Dr. Gott,** *I am starting your No Flour, No Sugar Diet and am confused as to what is "flour." I'm listing some ingredients in cereals and other items and I don't know if they are considered flour or not: whole barley, wheat flour, malted barley flour, corn flour, whole wheat, rice flour, corn bran, whole rye, whole oats, soy grits, whole hard red winter wheat, whole buckwheat, wheat bran, oat bran, rice, corn meal, and rolled oats.*

> **Dear Reader,** *I've tried to make my No Flour, No Sugar Diet as simple as possible. As I have stated before, if the word "flour" appears in the list of ingredients, the product should be avoided. Thus, in your letter, for example, "whole wheat" is acceptable, but "wheat flour" isn't.*

When I say "no flour," I'm not just referring to all-purpose flour, but rather flour of any kind. The point of my No Flour, No Sugar Diet is to replace the empty calories of highly refined foods with the nutrient-dense calories found in unprocessed foods. So when I say "no flour," I mean no all-purpose flour, but also no whole wheat flour or any product with the word flour in its ingredient list. Here are some flours to watch for as you read labels and peruse recipes:

all-purpose flour
pastry flour
cake flour

whole wheat flour
unbleached flour
rye flour
rice flour
brown rice flour
corn flour
barley flour

The not-so-sweet truth about sugar

Every day, the average American consumes 45 teaspoons of sugar, including cane and beet sugars, honey, molasses, maple syrup, and high fructose corn syrup. That's a whopping 675 empty calories. [From the U.S. Census Bureau's Statistical Abstract of the United States, 2002— http://www.census.gov/statab/www/]

Like processed flour, refined and concentrated sugars are made up of empty calories, offering your body little in the way of nutrition besides an energy rush that will be quickly followed by a crash, leaving you feeling fatigued and, paradoxically, hungrier than before. This is particularly true of cane sugar, beet sugar, and corn syrup, but also, to a lesser degree, of honey and other natural sweeteners.

Sugar goes by many different names, so even more than with flour, you need to be on the lookout for sugar in its many guises. When I say "no sugar," I mean regular table sugar, but I also mean anything labeled:

cane sugar
beet sugar
brown sugar
raw sugar
molasses
honey
evaporated cane juice

corn syrup (especially high fructose corn syrup)
maple syrup
brown rice syrup
glucose
sucrose

4

Enough About What You Shouldn't Eat— Let's Talk About What You Should Eat

Dear Dr. Gott, I am writing in reference to your No Flour, No Sugar Diet. Last year, I decided to prove to my wife that your diet absolutely would not work. She had been trying to get me to go on it for years. My first reaction, of course, was that I would have to give up eating so many things I like that it wasn't worth the small chance that I might actually lose a little weight. Once she told me all the things I could eat—including my favorite restaurant breakfast complete with hash browns and "Texas bacon," not to mention steak, baked potatoes with all the trimmings, and many other things—I decided I could suffer through this diet.

Well, to make a long story short, eight months after begin-ning your diet, and, quite honestly, eating like a horse, I have lost 46.5 pounds. I am retired and 68 years old. I went from 240 pounds to my present 193.5 pounds, and I feel great. I have not been at this weight for close to twenty years. Your No Flour, No Sugar Diet really does work. I feel guilty calling it a diet; I have never eaten so much and lost weight so easily.

Now that you understand the difference between "empty calories" and "nutrient-dense calories," you may have started to realize that cutting calories doesn't have to mean eating less food, feeling hungry all the time, or depriving yourself of the joys of eating delicious and satisfying meals. By focusing not on giving up your favorite foods but on replacing those empty calories with nutrient-dense ones, you can eat enough to remain full and satisfied even while you shed unwanted pounds.

A healthful diet is one that takes into account your body's need for foods from each of the three macronutrient food groups (carbohydrates, proteins, and fats), balances them in proper amounts, and utilizes foods that deliver a high ratio of nutrients to calories.

The ideal diet recommended by most nutrition experts is made up of about 50 percent carbohydrates, 35 percent protein, and 15 percent fat. In practice, this means each meal should include two to four ounces of lean protein (for instance, a piece of meat, chicken, fish, or tofu about the size of a deck of cards); a serving of whole grains or starchy vegetables (root vegetables, legumes, peas, corn, etc.,) about the size of your fist); and about two fists worth of non-starchy vegetables (leafy greens, squash, broccoli, cauliflower, etc.) or a combination of non-starchy vegetables and fresh fruit. The fat in your diet should come from cooking oils, like olive or canola oil, or from avocados, nuts, seeds, or low-fat dairy products.

To be sure you are eating the right balance of foods, try picturing your plate as a pie cut into four equal-sized pieces. One quarter should contain lean protein, one quarter should contain whole grains or starchy vegetables, and the remaining half should contain non-starchy vegetables or a combination of non-starchy vegetables and fresh fruit. This is a fail-safe method, provided you don't use gargantuan plates. Using the above visualization method, sticking with normal-sized dinner plates or smaller, will ensure that you don't overeat.

When choosing foods, the best way to ensure that you are getting the most nutrition out of the calories you consume is to modify your present diet to rely less on empty-calorie foods and more on the most nutrient-dense foods available.

Examples of nutrient-dense foods:

- Whole grains (including rolled oats, brown rice, whole wheat, barley, bulgur, quinoa, corn)
- Legumes (including peas, beans)
- Vegetables (including leafy greens, broccoli, cauliflower, squash, eggplant, asparagus, yams, tomatoes, carrots, cucumber, celery, artichokes)

• Fresh fruits (including apples, bananas, strawberries, raspberries, cherries, blueberries, pears, oranges, cantaloupe, honeydew melon, plums, peaches, apricots, nectarines)
• Lean meats
• Seafood
• Poultry (skinless)
• Soy products (tofu, soy nuts, etc.)
• Nuts and seeds
• Low-fat and nonfat milk products

Part II

A New Lifestyle
for a Better Life—
Tools to Help You Make
Healthier Choices

Dear Dr. Gott, Let me share an experience about weight loss. From the time I was a teenager, I never drank a diet soda, I drank the real thing. I've been fat since age 15 and I am now 67. During the intervening years, I have repeatedly lost—and regained—tremendous amounts of weight.

Finally after trying your No Flour, No Sugar Diet, I've begun to lose. I lost 45 pounds in the first three months. Under your instructions, I quit drinking regular soda, limited carbohydrate intake, and exercised regularly. The results are amazing. I feel better. This never happened before in 67 years of concentrated effort. I am committed to continuing your diet. Thank you for caring.

As you've heard from me before, if you want to lose weight steadily and consistently, eliminate from your diet foods that contain flour and/or added sugar and you'll easily cut out enough calories to lose the recommended one or two pounds a week.

Sounds easy, doesn't it? Well, it is easy, in that you don't have to weigh, count, or calculate anything or buy special food products or supplements. But changing lifelong habits always poses certain challenges. Before beginning a weight-loss endeavor, you must ask yourself one fundamental question: "Am I ready?"

Losing weight in a healthful way that will allow you to keep it off forever is a slow, sometimes taxing process. There will be many bumps in the road to achieving and maintaining your optimal weight. If you begin your program when you are really ready to commit to it, you are far more likely to be successful.

The first steps to achieving readiness are to accept that you are overweight, understand how you became that way, and realize the negative ramifications for your long-term health and lifestyle if you do not lose the excess weight. Remember that obesity is responsible for at least 300,000 deaths annually in the United States. In addition to serious health-related consequences, being overweight can also limit your mobility and energy levels, hindering your ability to participate in activities you enjoy—walking in the park, a game of tennis or volleyball, playing with your children or grandchildren. Between your physical health and your ability to enjoy life, there are endless reasons to lose the excess weight, but it's up to you to decide that it's worth the effort and to make the commitment to yourself.

This section offers tools and techniques you can use to ease your transition to a more healthful lifestyle. You'll learn how to make dietary choices that will help you achieve and maintain your goal weight and live a more active and fulfilling life.

5

Setting Realistic Goals

Dear Dr. Gott, I want to lose weight, so I tried your No Flour, No Sugar Diet. Success! I have lost 10 pounds in two months, but I am discouraged that I cannot slim down faster.

Dear Reader, As I have written before, dieters must be reasonable in their expectations. A loss of a pound a week is appropriate.

Any diet will result in an initial weight loss of several pounds a week due to "water weight." Fat holds fluid, so as the fat is lost, so is fluid—initially. Once this reaction runs its course, only fat is lost. So people who expect to lose two, three, or four pounds a week as a consistent pattern are being unreasonable.

You're doing fine. Stay on my diet. An average of a pound a week weight loss is an acceptable health goal. True, some weeks you may lose more (depending on your diet, activity, and water retention), some weeks less. But my expectation is an average of a pound a week. You didn't gain excess weight overnight, so you're not going to lose it overnight either.

Many people have a tendency to start on any program of change, including a weight-loss program, full of optimism and good intentions. Armed with a can-do attitude, they set the bar high, often so high it is impossible to reach. When they are unable to, say, lose 10 pounds the first week on their diet, they feel as though they have failed. They beat themselves up, which only leads to despair and low self-esteem.

Setting such unrealistic expectations for yourself is a symptom of a common self-defeating way of looking at the world that I call *dichotomous thinking*. This dichotomous thinking, in which you categorize things as either right or wrong, perfect or terrible, good or bad, etc., is a classic attitude problem that plagues many people on weight-loss programs. For instance, you might go six straight days meeting your caloric goals; then on the seventh day, you pig out and eat more calories than your program allows. The common response is, "I blew it, I'm off my program." The phrase "off my program" is a dichotomous view, indicating the incorrect conclusion that you are either perfect or terrible. Such dangerous despair from inevitable mistakes can lead to your giving up the diet.

Rather than expecting perfection of yourself, really think about what you can commit to right now. Setting realistic and attainable short-term goals will help you maintain your efforts and motivation. Make small changes in your diet, with the intention of building on those changes once they've become incorporated into your daily routine. Achieving one small goal will give you the confidence to set the bar a bit higher and reach the next realistic goal.

Remember that as many as 90 percent of people who lose weight quickly by severely restricting their caloric intake will gain the weight back—and often even more—as soon as they return to normal eating habits. Shedding pounds through rigorously restrictive dieting, rather than by learning to make wise food choices and exercising proper techniques for maintaining your ideal weight, is almost always ineffective as a lifelong weight management approach.

On the other hand, a slow, steady approach to weight loss will enable you to maintain your health and nourish your body, while still producing the results you desire. And you're more likely to keep the weight off over time. You'll have ups and downs, but that is to be expected. The weight loss will average out over time. Focus on setting and reaching attainable goals, and you'll be able to pat yourself on the back regularly for your small achievements, hence feeding your motivation to keep working toward the ultimate, larger goal of reaching your optimal weight.

Determining your goal weight

The first step in creating your diet plan is to determine how much weight you'd like to lose. Remember to be realistic in choosing your ultimate weight loss goal. You may have weighed 120 pounds in high school, but that doesn't mean it is an achievable weight for you now—or even a desirable one. Set your sights on a reasonable and achievable goal, a weight you feel you can actually achieve and be comfortable with.

Body Mass Index (BMI)

There are many ways to figure out what your optimal weight is. The Body Mass Index (BMI) is a widely accepted measure for determining if a patient is at an appropriate weight, overweight, or obese and whether or not the patient is at risk for developing certain obesity-related health complications.

The BMI measures your body weight in relation to your height and reflects how much of your body mass is made up of fat. To calculate your own BMI, you just need a calculator and to know your weight (in pounds) and your height (in inches). Your BMI is equal to your weight in pounds divided by your height in inches squared, then multiplied by 703. For instance, if you are 5 feet 4 inches tall (64 inches) and weigh 165 pounds, your BMI calculation would look like this: 165 divided by 4096 (64" x 64") multiplied by 703 = 28.3 BMI. See the chart on the next page.

What your BMI means

Underweight	Below 18.5
Normal	18.5 - 24.9
Overweight	25.0 - 29.9
Obese	30.0 and Above

A person with a BMI of 18.5 to 24.9 is considered to be at a healthful weight. A BMI of 25 to 29.9 is considered to be overweight, which carries moderate health risks. A BMI of 30 or higher indicates obesity and carries a serious risk of developing other health problems.

While BMI is not a perfect measurement, because it doesn't take into account certain extreme body types (such as serious athletes who have a lot of lean muscle mass or very short people, for example), it is considered a reliable way of assessing whether your weight is putting your health at risk.

When using BMI to determine your goal weight, aim for a weight that falls within the healthy range of 18.5 to 24.9. If you are starting out at a BMI of 32, however, it may be unrealistic to set a BMI of 22 as your goal. Start with a more achievable goal and, once you reach that goal and are able to maintain it for a while, revisit the BMI chart and perhaps

Body Mass Index Table

Height (inches)	Normal						Overweight					Obese										Extreme Obesity														
BMI	19	20	21	22	23	24	25	26	27	28	29	30	31	32	33	34	35	36	37	38	39	40	41	42	43	44	45	46	47	48	49	50	51	52	53	54
												Body Weight (pounds)																								
58	91	96	100	105	110	115	119	124	129	134	138	143	148	153	158	162	167	172	177	181	186	191	196	201	205	210	215	220	224	229	234	239	244	248	253	258
59	94	99	104	109	114	119	124	128	133	138	143	148	153	158	163	168	173	178	183	188	193	198	203	208	212	217	222	227	232	237	242	247	252	257	262	267
60	97	102	107	112	118	123	128	133	138	143	148	153	158	163	168	174	179	184	189	194	199	204	209	215	220	225	230	235	240	245	250	255	261	266	271	276
61	100	106	111	116	122	127	132	137	143	148	153	158	164	169	174	180	185	190	195	201	206	211	217	222	227	232	238	243	248	254	259	264	269	275	280	285
62	104	109	115	120	126	131	136	142	147	153	158	164	169	175	180	186	191	196	202	207	213	218	224	229	235	240	246	251	256	262	267	273	278	284	289	295
63	107	113	118	124	130	135	141	146	152	158	163	169	175	180	186	191	197	203	208	214	220	225	231	237	242	248	254	259	265	270	278	282	287	293	299	304
64	110	116	122	128	134	140	145	151	157	163	169	174	180	186	192	197	204	209	215	221	227	232	238	244	250	256	262	267	273	279	285	291	296	302	308	314
65	114	120	126	132	138	144	150	156	162	168	174	180	186	192	198	204	210	216	222	228	234	240	246	252	258	264	270	276	282	288	294	300	306	312	318	324
66	118	124	130	136	142	148	155	161	167	173	179	186	192	198	204	210	216	223	229	235	241	247	253	260	266	272	278	284	291	297	303	309	315	322	328	334
67	121	127	134	140	146	153	159	166	172	178	185	191	198	204	211	217	223	230	236	242	249	255	261	268	274	280	287	293	299	306	312	319	325	331	338	344
68	125	131	138	144	151	158	164	171	177	184	190	197	203	210	216	223	230	236	243	249	256	262	269	276	282	289	295	302	308	315	322	328	335	341	348	354
69	128	135	142	149	155	162	169	176	182	189	196	203	209	216	223	230	236	243	250	257	263	270	277	284	291	297	304	311	318	324	331	338	345	351	358	365
70	132	139	146	153	160	167	174	181	188	195	202	209	216	222	229	236	243	250	257	264	271	278	285	292	299	306	313	320	327	334	341	348	355	362	369	376
71	136	143	150	157	165	172	179	186	193	200	208	215	222	229	236	243	250	257	265	272	279	286	293	301	308	315	322	329	338	343	351	358	365	372	379	386
72	140	147	154	162	169	177	184	191	199	206	213	221	228	235	242	250	258	265	272	279	287	294	302	309	316	324	331	338	346	353	361	368	375	383	390	397
73	144	151	159	166	174	182	189	197	204	212	219	227	235	242	250	257	265	272	280	288	295	302	310	318	325	333	340	348	355	363	371	378	386	393	401	408
74	148	155	163	171	179	186	194	202	210	218	225	233	241	249	256	264	272	280	287	295	303	311	319	326	334	342	350	358	365	373	381	389	396	404	412	420
75	152	160	168	176	184	192	200	208	216	224	232	240	248	256	264	272	279	287	295	303	311	319	327	335	343	351	359	367	375	383	391	399	407	415	423	431
76	156	164	172	180	189	197	205	213	221	230	238	246	254	263	271	279	287	295	304	312	320	328	336	344	353	361	369	377	385	394	402	410	418	426	435	443

choose a new, lower goal. Even losing a small amount of weight—just 10 percent of your current body weight—will significantly lower your risk of developing obesity-related diseases.

If you are unsure about what an appropriate goal weight is for yourself, consult your physician. Work with your doctor to determine how much weight you need to lose to reduce your health risks, taking into consideration how much you are willing or able to alter your eating and exercise habits.

Embarking on a weight-loss program is a daunting task for many. If you've tried before to lose weight and failed, you may have a difficult time overcoming your belief that dieting is pointless. Try to think of your diet as a positive commitment to bettering yourself, rather than a pass/fail course in weight loss. Learning to make healthier food choices and incorporating more physical activity into your daily life will unquestionably lead to beneficial health consequences. And the truth is, if approached in the right way, you will most likely drop at least some, if not all, of your excess weight.

Write It Down: Keeping a Food Journal

For many people, overeating is simply a habit—you eat the foods you do when you do just because that is what you have always done. Replacing poor eating habits with good ones is an important key to achieving and maintaining your optimal weight. By changing the way you think about food and eating, you'll give yourself the tools you need to control your weight forever. But we all know that old habits are hard to break. The first step to changing a habit is to recognize the tendency in yourself and understand what drives it.

Keeping a food journal, a place where you record every morsel of food that passes your lips, helps you focus on what you are eating day to day. It is an excellent way to gain insight into when, what, and why you eat. You will no doubt be surprised at how much there is to learn about your eating patterns when you begin to document them.

Making the commitment to yourself to write down everything you eat has many benefits. First, it can help you curb your tendencies to overeat simply by making you acknowledge those choices in writing. You may find that simply knowing that you'll have to write down that bag of chips or giant chocolate chip cookie will deter you from eating it. Once you've got a few weeks' worth of data, you'll be able to examine them for eating patterns that you didn't even know you had. Maybe you overeat every Sunday when you have dinner with your sister. Or perhaps your trouble spots are weekdays when stress from work sends you scurrying to the candy machines several times a day. Whatever your bad habits are, a food diary will help you identify them by charting patterns that will jump out at you when you see them in black and white.

Getting started with your food journal

To start your food journal, I recommend that you buy a small notebook that can be tucked into your pocket or purse and carried with you wherever you go so that you can record what you eat immediately. You may be tempted to keep your journal on your computer, but if you don't record what you eat at the time that you eat it, you'll risk conveniently "forgetting" about it later when you have the time to update your journal. Many electronic organizers, however, have features that allow you to store notes, making them another convenient way to take your journal with you wherever you go.

What should you record in your journal? Everything and anything related to what, when, and why you eat every time you eat, every day. The value of the journal is lost if you only use it selectively. In order to identify eating patterns, you need to record every single piece of food or beverage (aside from water or other non-caloric beverages) you put in your mouth.

To make your journal a truly useful tool, you'll want to record not just what you eat, but how much, as well. Writing down "three slices of pepperoni pizza with extra cheese" or "one slice of thin-crust vegetable pizza" is a lot more informative than simply writing "pizza."

It is also important to record when you eat. Keeping track of this kind of information helps you to become aware of your eating patterns and to recognize where your pitfalls are. Do you tend to overeat when you're bored at work in the afternoons? Or maybe you munch mindlessly as you watch television at night. Once you know when you tend to overeat, you can develop a plan to curb those bad habits.

In addition to recording what, how much, and when you eat, it is also useful to keep track of how you are feeling, both physically and emotionally, when you eat. Each time you record a meal or snack in your journal, note how hungry you are. I like to use a scale of 1 to 5, with 1 being not at all hungry and 5 being on the brink of starvation. Note also your emotional state. Are you feeling happy? tired? sad? bored? lonely? stressed out? This information will help you recognize if you have a tendency to eat as a way of dealing with difficult or unpleasant emotions.

I recommend that you keep your food journal for a minimum of one full month to ensure that you get enough data to show any recurrent patterns. Many of my patients find journaling such a useful way to stay on top of their eating habits that they choose to continue their journals indefinitely, but you may find that a month of diligent journaling is all you need to gain a good understanding of your own patterns.

Look at the times when you eat the most, or are most likely to choose unhealthful foods, and see if you can discern any similarities between these instances. Using a highlighter can be useful in making these patterns really jump out at you.

Once you are able to recognize your personal eating patterns, you can begin to develop a plan to change them. For instance, if your food journal reveals a pattern of eating whenever you are confronted with a stressful situation at work, you can learn some relaxation exercises and practice them the next time you find yourself feeling overwhelmed. If you tend to comfort yourself with sweets when you're lonely, make a plan to call a friend or go somewhere where you can interact with others instead.

Remember, knowledge is power. Your food journal is a tool you can use to gain control over your eating habits rather than letting food control you. By keeping track of your eating habits and examining them for patterns and pitfalls, you'll learn to make better food choices that will allow you to control your weight for the rest of your life.

Some basic rules for keeping your food journal

Write everything down.

A piece of chocolate, a few pretzels, or a soda may not seem like much, but the calories from these small trespasses add up over time.

Do it now.

Record what you eat as soon as possible after eating it. Don't rely on your memory, which can be capricious.

Be specific.

If you ate a hamburger, write it down and be sure to include any extras like ketchup, mayonnaise, cheese, bacon, or a side of fries.

Estimate amounts.

Just recording the food you eat isn't enough to provide useful information. Record the size of your portions as well. If you had pizza, record the number of slices you had and include an estimate of the size of the pieces. If you had broccoli, make a note of whether it was one stalk or two cups.

Include details.

Extra information, such as whom you ate with, where you ate, and how you were feeling when you ate can be even more helpful than the specifics of what you ate when you are attempting to determine your eating patterns. Record as much information as possible about the circumstances surrounding your meals and snacks.

Sample food journal

Date: Monday 2/22/10

Food Eaten	Quantity	Time	Place	With	Cues	Hunger (1-5)	Emotions
Oatmeal	1½ cups	7:00	kitchen	alone	breakfast	4	sleepy
Banana	1						
Veggie soup	2 cups	12:15	lunchroom	coworkers	lunch	3	happy
Low fat cheese	2 ounces						
Apple	1 medium						
Almonds	1 ounce	3:30	office	alone	snack	2	starving
Chicken breast	4 ounces	7:00	kitchen	family	dinner	3	stressed
(with skin)							
Mixed greens	2 cups						
Vinaigrette	2 tablespoons						
Ice cream	½ cup						

33

Reading the Fine Print:
The Importance of Studying Food Labels

To be successful on the No Flour, No Sugar Diet, it is absolutely essential that you carefully read ingredient lists and nutrition labels when choosing foods. Reading the labels on the prepared and processed foods you buy is one of the most useful things you can do to control your diet.

Most packaged foods now carry nutritional information on their labels, listing the serving size and calories, fat, carbohydrate, protein, and sodium content per serving. Most important for my No Flour, No Sugar Diet, reading labels will help you spot hidden flour and sugar in foods you might not suspect contain them. Remember to watch for anything labeled "flour" or "sugar," including cane sugar, beet sugar, honey, maple syrup, corn syrup, molasses, glucose, and sucrose. You don't need to be overly stringent—for instance, frozen peas often contain small amounts of sugar, as do many frozen dinners, canned soups, and other foods that are generally acceptable on the diet—but do keep a watchful eye out for foods that contain significant amounts of these empty-calorie ingredients.

Calories per serving

While you don't need to count calories on the No Flour, No Sugar Diet, it is a good idea, at least in the beginning, to be mindful of serving sizes and calories per serving of the foods you eat. At first, you may even want to measure out your servings until you get an idea of what is meant by "one serving"—often it's a lot less food than you'd think. This practice can be quite helpful as you learn to make better food choices. By comparing calorie counts of different brands of the same food, for instance, you may find that simply substituting a new brand for an old favorite can cut unnecessary calories out of your diet.

Fat content

Dear Dr. Gott, My husband has been on your No Flour, No Sugar Diet for several weeks and has lost about 20 pounds. He finds the diet easy and enjoyable.

However, we have a disagreement as to the necessity of avoiding saturated fats. I say he should; he ignores me and continues to consume butter, cheese, potato chips, and mayonnaise. He thinks that as long as he avoids flour and sugar, he will lose weight and that's what counts. Can you resolve our problem?

Dear Reader, I think so.

My No Flour, No Sugar Diet is designed as a simple and inexpensive approach to weight loss. Although this diet does not prohibit fat, it—unlike the Atkins diet—does not encourage consumption of fat in any form, particularly the saturated variety. Actually, those people who endorse my diet usually end up eating less fat because, without toast, there's no butter; without pasta, there's less cheese, and so on.

So, in essence, my No Flour, No Sugar Diet should hopefully lead to a decrease in the consumption of fats. Even though I don't address this issue directly, I do not encourage dieters to substitute fat-rich edibles for the foods they have to avoid. Atkins did this and it is one of the major drawbacks of his diet.

Therefore, your husband's tendency to consume saturated fats is a separate issue that should be addressed aggressively if his cholesterol level is high (above 200 milligrams per deciliter), but in my opinion, can be put on the back burner if the level is 200 mg or less.

Weight loss is often favorably accompanied by a decrease in blood sugar and blood fat levels. If in your husband's situation this is not the case, some additional dietary restrictions may be in order.

You may also want to keep an eye out for fat content as you peruse labels. Again, my No Flour, No Sugar Diet doesn't require you to track or limit your fat intake, but, for a host of medical reasons, it's a good idea to limit the amount of fat—especially saturated and trans fats—in your diet. Remember a diet high in saturated fats, which come mostly from animal sources (meat and dairy products), can lead to elevated levels of LDL (the "bad" cholesterol) in the blood, increased risk of heart disease, and certain types of cancer. Trans fats have been shown to both raise LDL cholesterol while, at the same time, lowering levels of HDL (the "good" cholesterol). In 2006, the FDA will begin to require food manufacturers to list trans fat content on nutrition labels along with the other information about total fat as well as saturated fat content.

Another reason to watch your fat intake is simply that fat packs a lot of calories. In fact, while carbohydrates and proteins each have just 4 calories per gram, fats have 9 calories per gram. So, gram-for-gram, fat has more than twice the calories of either carbohydrates or protein. Ideally, your daily diet should contain no more than about 50 to 60 grams of fat, and most of those should be the unsaturated variety.

Cholesterol

Cholesterol is a fat-like substance found naturally in the human body. It is a necessary part of the body's metabolic processes and performs many essential functions, such as producing cell membranes and certain hormones. Your own body manufactures much of the cholesterol found in your bloodstream, while the rest comes from the foods you eat—primarily meats, poultry, fish, eggs, butter, cheese, and whole milk.

As I've mentioned previously, low-density lipoprotein (LDL), when present in the blood stream in excessive amounts, can clog your arteries and increase your risk of heart attack and stroke.

Reading nutrition labels is an important step in controlling the level of LDL in your blood, but you have to look at more than just the food's cholesterol content. Foods with high cholesterol content raise blood cholesterol, but saturated fat and trans fat in foods you eat raise blood cholesterol levels as well. Many "low-cholesterol" foods contain high levels of these fats, and thereby contribute to high blood cholesterol.

The American Heart Association recommends that people who do not suffer from coronary heart disease limit cholesterol intake from food to an average of no more than 300 milligrams per day. People with coronary heart disease should limit dietary intake of cholesterol to no more than 200 milligrams per day.

Dear Dr. Gott, After the holiday season, I was finally motivated to try your No Flour, No Sugar Diet (mainly omitting bread and desserts). In six months I had easily shed the extra 10 pounds. When I went for my six-month checkup, my astounded internist told me my cholesterol was 221 when it usually is about 270. Have any others reported a drop in cholesterol without drugs while doing the No Flour, No Sugar Diet?

Dear Reader, Because my No Flour, No Sugar Diet prohibits products such as bread and bagels, it automatically reduces the consumption of fat (butter on toast, cream cheese on bagels). As a result, this low-fat benefit can lead to significant reduction in the blood level of cholesterol. Thus, while not universal, your good fortune is relatively common. Keep up the good work.

Sodium

If you suffer from hypertension (high blood pressure) or have a family history of it, you'll also want to pay special attention to sodium content. Sodium is a mineral that helps to maintain your body's normal fluid levels and blood pressure, and it contributes to healthy muscle functioning. But the truth is, most of us consume a whole lot more than we actually need. There is ample evidence to suggest that many people at risk for developing high blood pressure—which can lead to heart disease, kidney disease, and stroke—may reduce their risk by limiting the amount of salt in their diet. The recommended limit for sodium in the diet is 2,400 milligrams. Paying attention to the sodium levels listed on food labels is a good way to keep your intake in check.

Fiber

Remember that fiber has no calories, yet it helps to keep you feeling full and satisfied. In addition, studies have shown that a diet low in saturated fat and cholesterol yet high in fiber may reduce your risk of certain cancers, diabetes, digestive disorders, and heart disease. "Soluble" fiber has been shown to help lower blood cholesterol, while "insoluble" fiber is an important aid in normal bowel function. Fiber is found in foods that come from plants, including fruits, vegetables, whole grains, and beans.

The U.S. Food and Drug Administration (FDA) recommends that a healthful diet include between 20 and 30 grams of fiber a day. The majority of your fiber intake will come from fresh fruits and vegetables. Reading labels will help you choose higher fiber versions of many common foods, such as breads and cereals.

8

Portion Control

Something really shocking has taken place in dining rooms and kitchens in this country over the past twenty years. Without most of us even realizing it, "normal" portions of food have doubled, tripled, even quadrupled in size. Look at this comparison of some common foods showing how many calories an average portion contained in the mid-1980s versus how many calories an average portion contains today:

Food	1984	2004
Blueberry muffin	210	500
Cheeseburger	333	590
Chicken Caesar salad	390	790
Popcorn	270	630
Cheesecake	260	640
Turkey sandwich	320	820
Soda	85	250
Chocolate chip cookie	55	275
French fries	210	610
Chicken stir fry	435	865
Spaghetti and meatballs	500	1025

(Source: Department of Health and Human Services, National Heart, Lung, and Blood Institute)

Thanks to this inflation of portion sizes, chances are you're eating a lot more than you realize. Recent studies have shown, for instance, that we often underestimate how many calories we consume each day by as much as 25 percent. If you dine in restaurants frequently or consume a lot of prepared meals, it's all too easy to lose track of just how much you're eating.

Learning to assess healthful portions—and limit yourself to those portions no matter where you eat—will help you enormously in achieving and maintaining your optimal weight. In fact, recent studies have shown that portion control may be the single most effective factor in healthy, long-lasting weight loss. You can continue to eat many of your favorite foods, provided you exercise some control and limit your servings to reasonable portions.

According to the United States Department of Agriculture (USDA), one serving is equal to:

1 slice of whole grain bread
½ cup of cooked rice
½ cup of mashed potatoes
½ cup of cooked or raw vegetables
1 cup of lettuce
1 small baked potato
1 medium apple
½ cup of berries
1 cup of yogurt or milk
1½ ounces of cheese
¼ pound hamburger patty

Here are some tips for visually assessing proper portions, without having to lug around a food scale or measuring cup:

A 3-ounce serving of meat is about the size of a deck of cards.
A 6-ounce serving of fish is about the size of a checkbook.
1 ounce of meat is about the size of a matchbook.
A 3-ounce serving of sliced lunchmeat is about the size of 3 CDs.
A 1-ounce serving of cheese is the size of a pair of dice.
1 cup of potatoes, rice, or cereal is about the size of a baseball.
½ cup of ice cream or frozen yogurt is about the size of 2 golf balls.
1 cup of fruit is about the size of a small fist.

Use the following tips and tricks to limit your portions:

Use smaller plates. With a smaller plate, you'll be less likely to serve yourself far more than you need. Plus, you'll feel like you're getting more.

Just eat half. The next time you're tempted by some of your favorite foods, try eating just half. Round out the meal with fresh veggies and fruit.

Take it home. Restaurant portions may be out of control, but that doesn't mean that you have to be. Just eat half of your serving and take the other half home. In addition to keeping you from overeating, this method enables you to enjoy the meal twice.

Read the label. When eating packaged foods, check the label to see what is considered a serving. You may be surprised at how small one serving really is. Measure out a single serving, and in the future you'll be able to eyeball the proper amount.

Don't eat out of the bag. When eating packaged foods—like popcorn or chips—put a single serving in a bowl rather than eating directly from the package.

Avoid all-you-can-eat buffets. If you have to eat at a buffet, look over the offerings first and decide which items you just can't live without. Fill your plate with reasonable servings, and don't go back for seconds.

9

Getting the Support You Need

Food and eating are integral to our culture. We celebrate births, engagements, weddings, new jobs, graduations, and anniversaries with feasts of all sorts. We go out to eat as a way to spend time with friends and loved ones. We break up long days in the office with fast food lunches with our coworkers. Eating together is one of our favorite social activities. It follows, then, that social support to help you stick to your weight loss program, change the way you approach food and eating, and reach your goal weight is an essential ingredient for success. In fact, research has shown that dieters who participate in weight loss programs that include weekly group support lose more weight and are more successful at keeping it off than people who try to go it alone.

Hearing about how others have struggled with the same weight loss challenges that confront you—and how they overcame them—can be extremely motivating. Other dieters can also provide advice, ideas, recipes, menus, and tips about local restaurants serving diet-friendly fare. A partner can motivate you to get out and exercise on those days that you'd rather just curl up on your couch in front of the television. A weight-loss buddy can also serve as your own personal cheering squad—pushing you to push yourself and celebrating your victories, big and small.

Where to find support

Since losing weight is dependent on changing the food choices you make every day, the ideal weight-loss partner is the person or people with whom you share the majority of your meals. If you live with others, see if you can get them to commit to eating a more healthful diet. Even if they don't need to lose weight, making better food choices will provide them with numerous lifelong health benefits. If you've got a friend who struggles with weight as you do, ask him or her to team up with you to conquer your dual weight problems once and for all.

Don't despair if you can't find a friend, family member, or loved one to partner with you.

If you're already committed to my No Flour, No Sugar Diet and are just looking for emotional support, consider nonprofit groups that offer support and education, but leave it up to you to develop an eating plan. Your local yellow pages or an Internet search can yield information about nonprofit weight loss organizations in your area.

Take Off Pounds Sensibly (TOPS) is a nonprofit organization that focuses on providing "a healthy, caring, and supportive approach to weight control at an affordable price." TOPS has been around for more than fifty years and offers education and a group-support environment to help people lose weight by making healthful lifestyle choices. For more information about TOPS, or to find a chapter near you, visit their website at www.tops.org.

Overeaters Anonymous offers a twelve-step program for recovery from compulsive overeating. OA is focused on providing a group support environment and tools to overcome compulsive eating behaviors. OA charges no dues or fees, although local chapters may request small donations to cover expenses. For more information, or to find an OA chapter near you, visit their website at www.oa.org.

Somewhat surprisingly, researchers have found that Internet-based support works just as well as face-to-face meetings. Many organizations, including TOPS, offer online versions of their programs. By becoming an online member, you have access to all of their materials and tools, including menu planners, calorie calculators, etc., and many also provide access to online forums where you can interact with other members and ask questions of diet and nutrition experts.

No matter where you find support for your weight-loss journey—at home, in your social circle, through organized groups, or online—it will help you reach your weight-loss goal. From providing information, advice, recipes, and ideas to offering emotional boosts and encouragement when you need them most, support of any kind is a valuable asset for anyone trying to make major lifestyle changes.

Don't Forget to Move:
The Importance of Exercise

More than 50 percent of adults in the United States do not get enough exercise to provide health benefits, and 25 percent of adults do not participate in any physical activity during their leisure time. Source: [Centers for Disease Control (cdc.gov)—US Physical Activity Statistics 2003 State Summary Data]

The best way to lose weight and keep it off is through a program that combines diet and regular physical activity. Increasing your level of physical activity will help you burn up the calories you eat, but exercise alone is a difficult path to weight loss since the amount of exercise you'd have to do to lose just one or two pounds by such means alone would be downright superhuman. If you cut down on your caloric intake while increasing your activity level, you will more easily achieve the negative calorie balance that will lead to weight loss.

Regular physical activity is crucial not just for achieving and maintaining your goal weight, but also for your general health and well being. Exercise helps you to build and maintain healthy bones, muscles, and joints, and it provides many proven benefits including a substantial reduction in the risk of death from the nation's leading cause of death—heart disease—as well as reducing the risk of diabetes, stroke, high blood pressure, and colon cancer. It lowers blood cholesterol levels and the risk of developing high blood pressure, and reduces blood pressure in people who suffer from hypertension. It even reduces feelings of stress, depression, and anxiety.

People who exercise regularly are less likely to be hospitalized than people who don't. They also visit the doctor less frequently and take fewer medications. For older people, exercise even reduces the likelihood of falling and fracturing bones while minimizing the pain caused by arthritis.

Do what you love

If you are a person who thinks you don't like to exercise, perhaps you just haven't found an activity you enjoy. I encourage you to explore numerous options until you find something that brings you real joy, in addition to keeping you physically fit. The more you enjoy your exercise program, the easier it will be to stick with it year in and year out. Lose the sedentary lifestyle forever by discovering a variety of physical activities that suit you. From walking and running to line dancing and rock climbing, there are activities that appeal to all personality types.

Many people who are not used to exercising regularly choose to start out by walking. Nearly anyone can take a walk. It doesn't require any special equipment, and it can be done just about anywhere. Begin by taking brisk walks around your neighborhood, through a local park, or even indoors on a treadmill while you watch television or return phone calls. If you choose walking as your exercise of choice, set both a distance goal and a frequency goal. Once you are meeting your original goal on a regular basis, up the ante and commit to walking farther or more often—or both!

If you're a highly social person, you may prefer exercise classes or even ballroom dance lessons. If you've got a streak of daredevil in you, you might try rock climbing at a local climbing gym or mountain biking at a nearby national or state park. Like popular music? Try a hip hop dance class. A nature lover? Hiking and backpacking will have you working up a sweat in the great outdoors. Got too much stress in your life? Yoga may be just the thing to calm your nerves and keep you centered. Do you enjoy being part of a team? How about joining a local softball, soccer, or hockey league? The possibilities are endless.

The following chart shows the per-hour calories burned performing a wide range of activities.

Physical Activity	Calories/Hour*
Stretching	180
Weight lifting (light workout)	220

Walking (3.5 mph)	280
Bicycling (up to 10 mph)	290
Light gardening/yard work	330
Dancing	330
Golf (walking and carrying clubs)	330
Hiking	370
Heavy yard work (chopping wood)	440
Weight lifting (vigorous effort)	440
Basketball (vigorous)	440
Walking (4.5 mph)	460
Aerobics	480
Swimming (slow freestyle laps)	510
Running/jogging (5 mph)	590
Bicycling (10 mph or greater)	590

*Calories/Hour for a 154-pound person

(*Source: USDA Dietary Guidelines for Americans, 2005*)

Keep trying different activities until you find one (or several!) that makes you look forward to your next opportunity to participate in it. If you get real enjoyment out of your exercise program, sticking with it will feel more like play than a chore.

If you need help getting and staying motivated, find an exercise buddy or two—walking or running mates, a dance partner, an exercise class colleague. If you need structure, take a class or hire a personal trainer or coach to get you started. If you're intimidated by a gym setting, get a few exercise DVDs or videos to get yourself in the groove.

If it has been years since you've done any sort of exercise and you're intimidated by the prospect of joining a gym or attending an exercise class, or are just plain afraid that you won't be able to complete a vigorous thirty-minute or sixty-minute exercise program, don't let that stop you. Any activity you feel comfortable with is better than no activity, so start with an easy ten-minute stroll around your neighborhood. Once you're able to do that easily, begin upping the frequency and duration of your sessions. Increase your walk to fifteen minutes, and try to go a little farther. Add five extra minutes per day to your walk and soon enough you'll be up to a good solid hour. Walk a little faster each day and try to cover more ground. To keep things interesting, vary your route from day to day.

Maybe you simply can't find a spare thirty to sixty minutes in your daily schedule to devote to exercise. That's okay, too. Even if you can't commit to a substantial exercise session, you can still get the recommended amount of exercise through smaller bursts of activity—perhaps ten minutes of stretching in the morning before work, a brisk fifteen-minute walk at lunchtime, a quick game of tag with the kids before dinner. Here are several ideas for fitting physical activity into your regular routine:

Walk or bike to work or school instead of driving
Park your car or get off the bus a few blocks from your destination
Opt for the stairs instead of the elevator or escalator
Play with your kids before or after work
Take the dog for a walk or a game of fetch in the park
Take up gardening or do-it-yourself home improvement
Invest in some hand weights or a treadmill or stationary bike and exercise while you watch television. Even stretching counts.

It takes up to six weeks for a regular activity to become a habit. Find an activity you like and commit to doing it regularly for six weeks. Chances are, by the time that six-week target rolls around, you'll be so used to your new routine that you won't even think of giving it up.

Dear Dr. Gott, I weigh 190 pounds and would like to lose 30 pounds. I walk an hour a day and do aerobics twice a week. Would I achieve more benefit from walking on a treadmill or lifting weights?

Dear Reader, I applaud your commitment to regular exercise. The type and extent of the activity is probably not as important as using your muscles regularly. As you've probably discovered, though, routine exercise can become boring. For this reason, I advise you to alter your routine. Lift weights one or two days a week, and use a treadmill two or three days. Intersperse this activity with brisk walking, swimming, cross-country skiing, biking, skating—whatever the season permits.

At the same time, avoid calorie-rich edibles that have little nutritional value: candy, sweets, refined sugar, junk food, and the like. You'll not only lose weight, but you'll feel better, too. Fitness and good health go hand in hand.

How much exercise is enough?

According to the Dietary Guidelines for Americans 2005, published by the USDA, every adult should engage in a minimum of thirty minutes of moderate physical activity per day to reduce the risk of chronic disease. To maintain a healthful body weight and avoid weight gain in adulthood, the USDA further recommends engaging in approximately sixty minutes of moderate- to vigorous-intensity activity most days, while simultaneously limiting caloric intake to within the recommended range for your gender, age, and activity level.

Exercise is beneficial to everyone—from small children to those in their late golden years. But how much is enough for you is difficult to say. People who are active in their younger years seem to enjoy ongoing exertion as they age. Some people continue to ski, run, and play tournament tennis into their eighties and nineties. On the other hand, a backhoe couldn't move some middle-aged folks from their favorite chairs in front of the television.

Exercise is a very individual matter. In general, you may safely exercise to the point of fatigue no matter what your age or level of physical fitness. Dangerous exercise consists of sudden strenuous exertion performed intermittently or on rare occasions. Most exercise-related problems arise when people begin an activity impulsively—engaging in sudden strenuous exercise without first warming up. Any exercise is good if it makes you feel good, but you have to be sensible. If you are basically sedentary, take it easy at first. Work into an exercise program gradually. It is always best to begin any new exercise program slowly.

Schedule time for exercise

All too often, people use the excuse of not having enough time as a reason not to exercise. If you want to have a fit, healthy body, exercise is not an option but a necessity. You don't skip sleeping or eating for lack of time, and you shouldn't skip exercising either. If exercise isn't already a part of you regular routine, you need to make time for it. This may mean eliminating some other activity, but more likely it means simply making a point to work exercise into your schedule. You may even find it helpful to write your planned exercise sessions into your appointment book and view these sessions as unbreakable appointments with yourself. If something comes up and you absolutely have to miss a planned exercise session, don't just cancel it. Reschedule it for another time. Remember, keeping your body fit is just as important as all of the other things you do.

Many medical experts recommend that if you are over forty, you should seek a special cardiac evaluation before beginning an exercise program. I think that if you are in relatively good health this is probably unnecessary, but if you are concerned, consult your doctor first.

Anyone can achieve physical fitness by incorporating cardiovascular conditioning, stretching exercises for flexibility, and resistance exercises or calisthenics for muscle strength and endurance into their lifestyle. Ultimately, your body is the best judge of how far you should push yourself. Listen to what it has to say.

11

Planning for Success

As with any project, having a solid plan mapped out ahead of time will help lead you down the road to success. A good diet plan takes into account not just how much weight you want to lose, but also your culinary likes and dislikes, any special dietary considerations such as allergies or food sensitivities, your schedule, and your social and family obligations. A well thought-out plan will also provide guidance on how to deal with the pitfalls and trouble spots that are likely to arise for anyone as he or she works through a weight-loss program. Determine a meal plan, make sure you have the foods you require in the house, and decide how you'll handle challenging situations. Then you'll be far less likely to grab unhealthful fast food meals on your way home from work.

First, clean house

The best advice I can give you about eating a healthful diet at home is to clean out your cupboards right away, getting rid of any products that don't fit with the No Flour, No Sugar Diet. Don't throw out nonperishable items—give them to a friend or donate them to a local food bank or homeless shelter. Remove all cookies, breads, pastries, pasta, and other foods containing flour. Dispose of all high-calorie sweetening products including sugar, molasses, maple syrup, honey, and corn syrup. Likewise, rid your cabinets, refrigerator, and freezer of any foods that are sweetened with sugar, honey, or other high-calorie sweeteners, including ice cream, pudding, peanut butter that has added sugar, and so on. Believe me, if you keep those foods in the house, no matter how good you are at sticking to the diet in the beginning, eventually you'll have a weak moment and go on a serious binge. Get those foods out of your house, and you won't even have to fight the temptation.

Shop for success

You may find it helpful to plan your meals several days or even a week ahead of time for one big shopping trip. Before you go shopping, write out a list of all the items you'll need to prepare the meals and snacks on your plan. Once you're in the market, stick to your list and be careful not to succumb to any urges to toss unhealthful impulse items into your cart. If you have only appropriate food at home, you're far more likely to stick to your diet.

Stock your no flour, no sugar pantry

Stocking your pantry with wholesome foods—sans flour and sugar, of course—may seem daunting at first, but having such foods on hand will help you enormously as you struggle with the day-to-day challenges of sticking to a diet.

The No Flour, No Sugar stock-your-pantry shopping list

Sweeteners
Artificial sweeteners, including Splenda and Equal
Fruit sweetener
Stevia

Dairy products
Skim milk
Low-fat, nonfat, or sugar-free yogurt
Low-fat or nonfat cheese
Eggs
Liquid egg substitute

Grains and cereals
Whole grain breakfast cereals that don't list flour or sugar in
    their ingredients
Oatmeal
Rice
Barley
Quinoa
Bulgur
Polenta
Corn tortillas (made with corn rather than "corn flour")

Meat, fish, poultry

Lean lunch meats (sliced turkey breast, turkey ham, etc.)
Skinless poultry (white meat preferred)
Fish, including tuna, salmon, cod, trout, etc.
Shellfish, including shrimp, crab, scallops, clams, mussels
Pork tenderloin
Extra-lean ground beef
Ground turkey

Beans and legumes

Beans, dried or canned, including kidney beans, lentils, chickpeas
Tofu
Soy-based vegetarian meat substitutes, including veggie pepperoni, veggie burgers, tofu hot dogs, soy-based sausages

Fruits and vegetables

Lettuce leaves (for salads and as wrappers)
Celery
Endive
Leafy greens, including lettuce, spinach, kale, and cabbage
Brussels sprouts
Mushrooms
Broccoli
Cauliflower
Squash, including zucchini, acorn, butternut, pumpkin
Radishes
Green beans
Peppers, including red, green, and yellow bell peppers
Asparagus
Tomatoes
Eggplant
Avocados
Fresh herbs, including basil, mint, and oregano
Onions
Apples
Peaches
Nectarines
Apricots
Figs

Cherries

Berries (raspberries, blueberries, blackberries, strawberries,)

Grapes

Melons (cantaloupe, honeydew, watermelon)

Oranges

Bananas

Quick meals and snacks

Broth-based soups that don't contain noodles—vegetable, tomato, beef barley, mushroom, miso

Hummus

Salsa

No-sugar-added peanut butter or other nut butters

Toasted nuts, especially almonds, pistachios, and soy nuts

Dill pickles

Edamame (soy beans in the pod)

Condiments

Pickle relish (be sure to check the label for sugar)

Mustard (not honey mustard or other sweetened varieties)

Salad dressings (check for sugar content)

Low-fat or nonfat sour cream

Low-fat or nonfat mayonnaise or soy-based mayonnaise

Soy sauce

Hot pepper sauce

Salsa

Fruit juice-sweetened jams and fruit preserves

Balsamic vinegar

Sweet treats

Sugar-free candy (check for flour and watch out for high fructose corn syrup and other high-calorie sweeteners)

No-sugar-added ice cream and frozen yogurt

Sugar-free pudding made with skim milk

Sugar-free Jello

Cooking fats

Olive oil, canola oil, sunflower oil, safflower oil

Butter (use sparingly)

Having plenty of healthful food options on hand will make it easy for you to eat delicious and satisfying food while still sticking to your diet goals.

Who has the time to stick to a diet? You do!

You probably have to meet numerous challenges every day. The list may include working long hours, excruciating commutes, chauffeuring kids around to their myriad activities, all the while keeping up with the housework and finding the time to shop for and prepare well-balanced meals—not to mention squeezing in an exercise session.

But lack of time is no excuse for failing to make healthful choices. Planning ahead of time is the best way to ensure that even when you're pressed for time and stressed to the gills, you'll be able to choose foods that support a nutritious lifestyle, to get the exercise you need, and to continue on the road to your goal weight.

Prepackaged meals are a great convenience item, even when you are watching what you eat. Fortunately, there are more and more prepared foods available in our supermarkets, and, as long as you choose wisely, these can be lifesavers as you try to fit healthful eating into your busy life. The important thing is to read labels and choose foods that are nutritionally well-balanced, low in fat and calories, and, of course, don't contain flour or sugar. In the beginning, you may need to spend a little extra time in the market weighing your choices, but eventually you'll learn to tell, at a glance, which foods are nutritious and within your calorie limits and which are not. Having a few of these prepared foods in your freezer is a great fallback tactic for those days when you just don't have the time to prepare a full meal yourself.

If you like to cook, make-ahead meals are also a great way to ensure you'll always be able to make appropriate choices. In the recipe section later in the book, I include several recipes for snacks and meals that can be made ahead and stored until hunger strikes.

Plan to snack

Snacking throughout the day is a great way to stave off serious hunger pangs, and it may actually keep you from overeating at mealtimes. A couple of well-planned low-calorie snacks during the day can help ensure

Treating hypertension (the symptom) while ignoring the underlying disease is sometimes inescapable but will usually reduce the negative consequences of hypertension and prolong life.

Busting Myths and Avoiding Negative "Remedies"

Dear Dr. Gott, A man and his wife who are close friends of mine are trying to live on vitamins only—no food to speak of. Only when extremely hungry do they make a sandwich or order in fast food or a pizza. Vegetables, meat, fish, and fruit are basically avoided. Isn't this practice an open invitation to nutritional deficiencies? They refuse to accept this view.

Dear Reader, A diet made up merely of vitamins with periodic binge eating will probably not satisfy their nutritional requirements in the long run. While I hesitate making any specific predictions, a diet that is nutritionally deficient could, sooner or later, adversely affect your friends' immune systems as well as contribute to a variety of ills such as anemia and heart disease (from inadequate protein intake). While the couple may not listen to you, show them my response to your question. Or, better yet, urge them to review their dietary plans with a physician.

I may sound like a broken record, but this point bears repeating: the only way to lose weight is to eat fewer calories and/or burn more through physical activity. Myths abound about how to lose weight faster and more easily, but the bottom line is that there is no magic pill that will make the pounds drop off effortlessly without serious risks to your overall health and well being.

Appetite suppressants

Dear Dr. Gott, I have considered taking an over-the-counter medicine to lose weight. The tablets contain phenylalanine. Does this ingredient have any side effects or hazards?

Dear Reader, *Phenylalanine is an amino acid needed for good health. It is plentiful in many foods, including dairy products. It is harmless and will cause no side effects.*

If phenylalanine is the active ingredient in the product, you're being taken for a ride; the amino acid will not affect your weight. Read the label again and check out the other components. Many nonprescription diet pills contain phenylpropanolamine (PPA), an appetite suppressant that should not be taken by patients with diabetes, thyroid disorders, or irregular heartbeats. In addition, the substance often causes jitteriness, nervousness, and insomnia.

Desperate to lose weight, some dieters will turn to everything from mild stimulants, like the above-mentioned PPA, to dangerous drugs for weight loss: ephedra, methamphetamines (speed, Ritalin, Adderal), cigarettes (for the appetite suppressing properties of nicotine), and even narcotics. While these methods may produce dramatic weight loss, the long-term health risks far outweigh the benefits.

Like weight loss methods that severely restrict food intake, the use of appetite suppressants is not a viable solution for maintaining your ideal weight in the long run. Because they dampen your drive to consume food, you'll lose weight simply because you are eating fewer calories, but you may also be missing out on important nutrients that keep your body strong and healthy. Furthermore, once you stop taking the appetite suppressants, you'll likely gain back any weight you lost, because you didn't learn to change your behavior to sustain an ideal weight.

To make matters worse, many of these compounds have dangerous side effects, including anxiety, sleeplessness, irregular heartbeat, respiratory disorders, blood clots, liver damage, and addiction. While terribly alluring, these drugs are, at best, ineffective over the long haul and, at worst, downright dangerous.

I discourage the use of appetite suppressants of any kind, as they do not help people maintain their ideal weight. Studies have shown that more than nine out of ten people who lose weight by using appetite suppressants will regain the lost pounds within a year or two. Once you stop taking the appetite suppressants, you usually gain back the weight you lost because you didn't learn to change your behavior patterns to sustain an ideal weight. Far more effective for long-term weight loss and weight maintenance is to adopt a healthful eating pattern that can be sustained throughout a lifetime.

Laxatives and diuretics

In the never-ending quest to be thin, many people turn to laxatives and diuretics to help them lose weight or keep it off. Both laxatives and diuretics work primarily by causing the body to excrete excess water. The weight lost is simply water weight, not body fat, and is quickly regained once the body is rehydrated. Misuse of these substances can cause dehydration, long-term damage to the digestive tract, and deficiencies in important nutrients—including calcium, potassium, magnesium, and zinc.

Dear Dr. Gott, I'm a compulsive over-eater. Does dieting to control weight followed by binge-eating have any effect on my overall health?

Dear Reader, Recent studies have shown that overweight people who lose and gain weight cyclically are at greater risk of health problems (such as heart disease) than are stout folks who maintain constant weights.

Therefore, unless you're so motivated to lose that you're willing to stick to a consistent diet, I recommend that you swear off the diet-binge-eating cycles. You'll feel better about yourself and life will certainly be less complicated for you.

Check with your doctor about this to make sure that you don't have an undiagnosed ailment, such as diabetes, that may be contributing to your problem. Also, because of your addictive pattern of eating, you might consider counseling. Compulsive overeating is a form of substance abuse.

"Natural" weight loss aids

There is a common misconception that if a weight loss aid or dietary supplement is "natural," it must be safe. But since the only natural way to lose weight is to eat less and exercise more, it follows that even so-called "natural" weight loss aids are just as ineffective, gimmicky, and unsafe as "unnatural" ones.

Apple cider vinegar

Proponents of apple cider vinegar as a weight loss aid claim that pectin, a soluble fiber present in the vinegar, binds to cholesterol and removes it from the body. Unfortunately, there is simply no scientific evidence to support such a claim. Apple cider vinegar is just vinegar.

Chitosan

Chitosan is a dietary fiber derived from the shells of shellfish. Producers of the supplement claim that it binds to fat and cholesterol contained in the food we eat, preventing it from being absorbed by the body. Taken in large quantities, though, chitosan has been shown to interfere with absorption of fat-soluble vitamins and may cause gas, bloating, and diarrhea. Furthermore, research has shown that chitosan supplements are only associated with weight loss when they are combined with a low-fat, low-calorie diet.

Chromium supplements

Makers of chromium supplements contend that the pills serve to lower blood sugar, reduce body fat, control hunger, reduce cholesterol and triglyceride levels, and increase muscle mass. Certain forms of chromium, however, including the popular chromium picolinate, have been linked with adverse side effects including anemia, memory loss, and DNA damage. Research has provided mixed evidence in regard to chromium's effectiveness as a weight loss aid.

Diet teas

Diet teas are dietetic primarily because (like all plain teas) they're calorie-free. Some contain diuretic or stimulant herbs, which cause weight loss either by causing the body to excrete fluids or by suppressing the appetite. These herbal cocktails are at best ineffective and at worst can be extremely harmful in large quantities. Stimulant teas, in theory, cause weight loss by suppressing appetite but they carry risks similar to other appetite suppressants—nervousness, headaches, and sleeplessness. Examples of stimulant ingredients include ephedrine, ma huang, kola nut, and guarana.

Diuretic weight loss teas, like diuretic tablets, cause weight loss by depleting the body of fluids. By causing excess water loss, these teas may also reduce levels of important minerals such as potassium, which can lead to serious health risks. Common ingredients found in such teas include senna, locust plant, angustofolia, cassia angustofolia, cascara, and buckthorn.

Fiber supplements

While fiber found in foods such as fresh fruits and vegetables can help you lose weight by filling you up without added calories, thereby helping you to consume less food, fiber supplements don't do anything to promote weight loss directly and can have harmful effects on the digestive system if used to excess.

Glucomannan (konjac) and guar gum

Glucomannan (konjac) and guar gum are vegetable fibers that expand and become gel-like in the stomach, allegedly decreasing appetite. Glucomannan can cause problems because it may expand in the throat or esophagus and cause choking, obstruction, and asphyxiation.

Grapefruit

Grapefruit in and of itself does nothing to increase weight loss or metabolism. Many grapefruit-diet pills contain the over-the-counter stimulant and appetite suppressant phenylpropanolamine (PPA), which can cause anxiety, hypertension, and palpitations.

Green tea extract

Green tea extract pills contain polyphenols, powerful antioxidants that may help lower cholesterol and triglycerides. Since green tea naturally contains caffeine, use of these supplements may suppress the appetite but may also cause nervousness or insomnia.

Growth-hormone releasers

Human growth hormone (HGH) is a substance secreted by the pituitary gland that promotes growth during childhood and adolescence. Levels of the hormone naturally decrease as we age. Proponents of "growth hormone releasers," supplements that are purported to stimulate the release of HGH, assert that increased levels of HGH in the blood will reduce body fat and build muscle. Scientific evidence for such claims, however, is thin. These supplements are expensive, generally believed to be ineffective, and potentially harmful.

Kelp

Kelp, a type of seaweed, has been touted as a weight loss supplement on the basis that it is a rich natural source of iodine, which helps the thyroid gland regulate the body's metabolic rate. The truth of the matter is that you undoubtedly get enough iodine in your daily diet, and supplemental doses of this mineral are superfluous.

Lecithin

Lecithin is a natural component of many foods, including egg yolks, soybeans, grains, wheat germ, fish, legumes, yeast, and peanuts. Producers of lecithin supplements claim that they encourage weight loss by breaking down fat so that it can be flushed from the body. There is no scientific research that proves this to be true, and a healthful diet will provide all the lecithin a person needs anyway, making supplements unnecessary.

Lipotropic "fat burners"

Lipotropic substances prevent fat accumulation in the liver, but there is no scientific evidence that they promote weight loss.

Meal-replacement liquids

Meal-replacement liquids are variations on liquid-protein crash diets. They don't alter eating habits that lead to overweight, and they can cause imbalances, deficiencies, and constipation.

Spirulina

Spirulina, a type of algae, is said to suppress appetite, but this claim has yet to be scientifically proven. Spirulina does contain certain essential nutrients, including protein, and is considered an acceptable part of a varied diet. Taken in large quantities as a weight loss aid, however, it may lead to toxic levels of certain nutrients.

Starch blockers

The FDA banned bean derivatives known as starch blockers until they could be proven safe and effective—and there's no proof yet. These supplements can cause serious digestive problems.

St. John's Wort

Proponents of this herbal supplement claim that it suppresses the appetite, but the FDA has not found sufficient evidence to support this claim. Side effects may include gastrointestinal distress, tiredness, and sleeplessness.

Vitamin B$_6$

Vitamin B$_6$, also known as pyridoxine, is believed to aid in releasing energy from the food we eat. It is found in ample quantities in potatoes, oats, meat, fish, eggs, beans, bananas, avocados, nuts, and seeds. Vitamin B$_6$ may have some mild diuretic effects, but in excessive quantities it can cause numbness and nerve damage.

Just say no to extreme diets

If you are overweight, losing excess pounds is an important step in improving your present health and protecting you from serious illness down the road. As important as it is, though, to shed your extra weight, it's equally important to ensure that you consume the essential nutrients you need. Extreme diets, those that lure you with claims of instant weight loss with little effort, often do more harm than good.

Dear Dr. Gott, I have relatives who have gone crazy over a liquid-diet drink. They plan to consume the beverage for the rest of their lives to maintain a higher energy level and still lose weight. Is there any hope for the rest of us who remain firm believers in the value of regular exercise and prudent eating habits?

Dear Reader, There are many diet programs and weight-reduction plans available today. Because they are so restrictive, they do enable people to shed unwanted pounds over the short haul. However, they're almost impossible to follow for any length of time. Thus any initial weight loss is customarily short-lived; the pounds invariably reaccumulate when the person eventually "relaxes" and begins eating as before. The resulting yo-yo effect (cycles of loss and gain) is unhealthful.

In my view—and in the opinion of experts—it makes more sense to exercise regularly and adopt sensible, long-term dietary modifications with which a person feels comfortable. For example, most stout people can lose weight (and keep it off) by reducing dietary fat, moderating alcohol intake, and avoiding foods that contain added sugar and flour.

Low-carb/high-protein diets can lead to a host of health problems

Finally, the backlash against the low-carb craze has begun to set in. For years, it seemed practically the whole world had gone crazy with carbophobia. Many people lost weight following extreme low-carb diets like the Atkins Diet but at what cost to their long-term health? Low-carbohydrate diets can cause several health concerns over time.

First and foremost, by encouraging an intake of excessive amounts of animal protein, cholesterol, and saturated fat and limiting the intake of high-fiber foods like fruits, vegetables, and whole grains, many low-carb diets increase the risk of high cholesterol, hypertension, and heart disease.

A diet high in protein and fat and low in fiber, vegetable protein, and whole grains may also lead to an excess of uric acid, which in turn can lead to kidney stones and gout—a terribly painful form of arthritis that usually affects the big toe.

Consumption of excessive amounts of dietary protein causes calcium to be excreted by the liver, which can lead to osteoporosis, a disorder in which bone calcium is reduced, resulting in abnormally brittle bones. Inadequate fiber in the diet can also lead to osteoporosis by decreasing the body's ability to absorb calcium.

A limited intake of fiber-rich fruits, vegetables, whole grains, and legumes increases the risk of constipation, as well as the risk of colon cancer, diverticulitis, Crohn's disease, hemorrhoids, and irritable bowel syndrome. A diet high in whole grains, legumes, fruits, and vegetables—all rich in soluble and insoluble fiber—lowers these risks.

Extremely low-calorie diets may be making you fat

It seems paradoxical, but drastically limiting your caloric intake to a level below your basic caloric needs can actually stymie your weight loss efforts. When your body doesn't get enough calories, it goes into starvation mode, conserving energy by slowing down your metabolism. This can make it progressively more difficult to lose weight and keep it off.

When deprived of the fuel it needs to perform all of its daily functions, your body will begin to break down muscle tissue, causing a release of nitrogen into your system. This nitrogen is quickly washed away by water released by the cells. The result is an immediate reduction of the amount of water in your body, hence a sudden and notable loss of pounds. But this loss is short-lived. Water weight will be regained immediately once you rehydrate your system.

To make matters worse, the loss of muscle ultimately results in a slower resting metabolism. Muscle tissue burns calories, so the more muscle you have, the more calories you burn even when you are at rest. Any reduction in muscle mass causes a reduction in the number of calories your body burns each day. If you lose muscle and continue to eat the same number of calories, you will gain weight rather than lose it over the long term. Since most of us are unable to maintain extremely low-calorie diets for any length of time, we'll quickly regain lost weight. To make matters worse, our metabolisms are now slower since we've lost muscle mass. In order to maintain our weight, we must consume even fewer calories than before we started dieting.

A healthful diet, one that includes enough calories to fuel and nourish your body adequately, combined with an exercise program designed to burn calories and build muscle mass will enable you to lose weight and keep it off.

Do you really need "super foods"?

The health and fitness media have gone crazy lately over *super foods*, edibles high in certain nutrients that are touted as powerhouse disease-preventers. No doubt you've heard about red wine's ability to protect against heart disease, blueberries' cancer preventing antioxidants, and soy's usefulness in relieving menopausal symptoms. These foods are thought to prevent disease because they contain phytochemicals and antioxidants. You may be tempted to focus on one particular food in your diet in an attempt to capitalize on these benefits, but leading nutrition researchers warn that focusing on individual foods to the exclusion of others may fail to deliver the desired health benefits, and in some cases may actually increase certain risks.

According to scientific research, nutrients tend to work as a team, rather than individually. By focusing on a single food in the hopes of reaping the benefit of a certain nutrient, you may unwittingly create nutrient imbalances that actually increase your risk of disease. For instance, consuming too much iron can limit the body's ability to absorb zinc, a nutrient essential for healthy immune functioning. Too much vitamin A may cause your body to excrete vitamin D, which is necessary for getting calcium to your bones.

Repeated studies have shown that consuming a wide array of fruits and vegetables can reduce the risk of diabetes, heart disease, stroke, and certain cancers. But most of this research supports the idea that it is the variety and combination of nutrients that provide benefits rather than any one specific nutrient on its own. A diet that includes an array of plant foods—fruits, vegetables, legumes, and whole grains—is your best bet both for maintaining an appropriate weight and ensuring that you get sufficient doses of important disease-fighting nutrients.

Back to basics

The more the medical establishment learns about diet and nutrition, the clearer it seems that the best way to maintain a healthful weight is simply to eat a varied diet that is low in saturated fat, cholesterol, and empty calories, and includes a wide range of nutrient-dense fruits, vegetables, and whole grains. Eliminate junk food, snack on raw vegetables, switch from sugar to no-calorie sweeteners, and exercise regularly. By sticking to my No Flour, No Sugar Diet, you'll continue to get all the nutrients you need, while easily cutting enough calories to lose excess weight and keep it off—and, most important, you won't increase risks to your long-term health.

Staying on Track

Dear Dr. Gott, *My father told me about your No Flour, No Sugar Diet and it worked really well for me. I lost 15 pounds in about a month and a half. I like this diet better than the Atkins Diet because it's a lot easier and it feels better on my body. When I was on Atkins, I could feel my arteries getting clogged and I always felt short of breath. I've never felt that way before.*

I'm not very overweight. My goal is only another 10 to 15 pounds. My problem is that I'm stuck. I've been stuck for a couple of weeks now. I wanted to know how I could get over this hump. My mother and sister have the exact same problem. They, too, have lost about 15 pounds each. Is there anything we can do? Are there more details to the diet we need to know about? Your answer will be greatly appreciated.

Dear Reader, *People on any diet will not lose weight every week; sometimes the weight-loss rate flattens out for a period of time, what you properly termed "the hump."*

Don't be discouraged. Continue the diet, modify your portions, and keep exercising. Eventually you will shed those unwanted pounds.

By design, my No Flour, No Sugar Diet is simple and easy to fit into your life. In these pages, I've provided tools to help you design and implement a practical and balanced meal plan, improve your level of physical activity, and more—all as part of a well-designed plan to help you achieve and maintain your optimal weight. But even with all this careful planning, losing weight is a slow and often arduous process. Getting started may be difficult, but staying motivated and on track can sometimes feel like a near-impossible endeavor. Having backup plans and predetermined responses to the inevitable challenges will help you stay the course and reach your goal.

Dining out

Eating in restaurants is one of the biggest challenges for dieters, but don't despair. You can continue to enjoy eating out while on the No Flour, No Sugar Diet. All it takes is a little extra thought and planning.

First off, if you know you'll be dining at a certain restaurant, it's a good idea to check out the menu before you go. Many restaurants now have web sites. Try doing an Internet search for the restaurant you plan to go to. If you're lucky, you'll find a web site that includes the restaurant's menu. Look it over and decide ahead of time what you'll order. This will prevent you from making an impulsive, and possibly poor, choice while you're sitting ravenous in the restaurant.

If you can't find a web site, call the restaurant. Explain that you are on a special diet and ask what dishes they serve that do not contain flour or sugar. Ask, too, if the kitchen will accommodate substitutions. For instance, will they substitute steamed vegetables or salad for pasta? This will save you from any potential embarrassment or awkwardness that might arise from grilling your server while your dining companions sit waiting to order.

A few basic rules can help you avoid dishes containing flour and/or added sugar:

Ask questions! Your waitperson can give you information about ingredients not listed on the menu. If he or she doesn't know the answer, request that the chef be consulted.

Make substitutions. If a dish comes with a side of pasta, ask your server if steamed vegetables, a green salad, fresh fruit, or brown rice can be substituted.

Ask for croutons to be left off your salad.

Tell your server not to bring a bread basket to your table. If your companions want bread, ask that it be moved to the far side of the table from you.

Avoid dishes that are "breaded" or "battered," as these most likely contain flour.

Skip pasta dishes or any dish containing noodles (chow

mein, beef Stroganoff, chicken noodle soup, etc.).

Pass on anything with a crust—pot pie, quiche, tart, and fruit pies all contain flour (and dessert versions also contain sugar).

Ask for sandwiches and burgers to be served in lettuce leaves instead of bread, rolls, or buns.

In Mexican restaurants, skip the tortilla chips and ask if corn tortillas are made with corn flour or just corn. If they are made with just corn, they are acceptable. Flour tortillas and tortillas made with corn flour should be avoided.

In Italian restaurants, choose risotto, meat, fish, or poultry dishes instead of pasta or pizza.

In Chinese restaurants, skip anything with a sauce described as "sweet" (sweet and sour, sweet and spicy, etc.) as these contain sugar. Other sugary sauces to avoid include lemon, orange, hoisin, and plum. And, of course, skip noodle-based dishes like chow mein and dumplings wrapped in flour-based wrappers (egg rolls, pot stickers, etc.).

In Thai restaurants, avoid the sweet chili dipping sauce and peanut sauce, both of which are made with sugar. Also skip rice noodle dishes like Pad Thai, spring rolls, and summer rolls, as their wrappers are made from rice flour.

In Japanese restaurants, steer clear of teriyaki sauce, which is loaded with sugar, and skip any noodle-based dishes like udon or soba noodle soup.

Skip dessert. If you really need something to finish off the meal, order a hot cup of decaffeinated coffee or tea and sweeten it with Splenda or another no-calorie sweetener.

Watch your portion size. No matter what you order, if you are served an excessively large portion, ask for a take-out box, and put half of your dish in it before you even start eating. That way you won't be tempted to eat more than you need.

Don't be shy about asking questions or making special requests. You should be able to find acceptable dishes on just about any restaurant menu. By choosing wisely and substituting acceptable side dishes for unacceptable ones, you'll be able to enjoy dining out and still stick to the No Flour, No Sugar Diet.

Sticking to the diet when your family isn't on it with you

It can be especially challenging to stick to a new eating plan if the people closest to you are still enjoying your old habits. To be able to change your lifestyle habits while confronted with temptations and surrounded by poor examples requires an extra level of commitment on your part. Remember that you are doing this for yourself, and are resolving to set an example for others. In time, your loved ones may be so impressed by your weight loss and the gains you've made in terms of health and fitness that they'll ultimately want to follow your lead. In the meantime, explain to them that this is important to you, and, while you can't force them to go on the diet with you, ask that they respect your needs. Ask them to consume junk food outside of the home, rather than keeping it stocked in the kitchen cabinets where it will create an unnecessary temptation for you.

Preparing for holidays, vacations and special occasions

Even if you've completely overhauled your lifestyle and eating habits, certain events threaten to derail your best efforts. Holidays, birthdays, weddings, and vacations don't just invite overeating, they often actually center around it. To make matters worse, during the busy holiday season or when you're on vacation, you're less likely to stick to your exercise routine. But there's good news. My No Flour, No Sugar Diet is designed to be flexible enough to allow for occasional transgressions. The key is to plan ahead.

Prepare for holidays, vacations, and special occasions by dieting stringently in advance. If you've continued to consume potatoes, rice, and alcohol, for instance, try cutting these from your diet for a week or two before the event. By being extra-stringent in anticipation of special occasions, you can build up "credits" that you can spend on the big day. If you've been diligent about your diet in the days leading up to the event, overdoing it a bit won't destroy all your efforts. Just be sure to limit your loosening of the reins to the occasion, and get right back on the program the next day.

You've gone on an unanticipated binge—now what?

First of all, don't panic. Remember that the beauty of the No Flour, No Sugar Diet is that it is flexible. So you went crazy and pigged out on pasta and chocolate cake. Just be extra diligent over the next few days. If your weight has crept up a bit, stick to the strictest version of the diet until it comes off again.

15

Keep It Off:
Maintaining Weight Loss
Once You Have Reached Your Goal

The biggest problem with most fad diets is that, while they may be successful at generating initial weight loss, that loss is nearly impossible to maintain over time. Because these diets tend to be either overly restrictive or simply too complicated to maintain as an ongoing part of a normal life, dieters ultimately return to their old eating habits and regain all of the weight they lost—and often even more. Remember, as I have said before, as much as 90 percent of people who lose weight quickly on fad diets regain all of that weight.

Unlike typical fad diets, my No Flour, No Sugar Diet is not just a weight loss program, but a healthful way of eating that can help you to maintain your optimal weight throughout your life. It doesn't require you to cut out any food group entirely, subsist on expensive specialty products, or restrict your caloric intake so severely that you can only do it safely for short periods of time. Instead, it teaches you to make healthful choices every day that add up to a nutritious way of eating that will keep you fit and healthy for many years to come.

I designed the program to be flexible enough to suit people with many different needs. So whether you're at the beginning of your weight loss journey with 100 pounds or more to lose, or simply want to maintain the healthful weight you've already achieved, this program will work for you.

Weekly weigh-ins

Weighing yourself once a week—ideally at the same time of day using the same scale—is an extremely important element in the continuing success of people who have used my No Flour, No Sugar Diet. This is such a simple technique that I'm shocked more diet plans don't include this sort of home monitoring as a measure of continued success. The information gained from such weekly weigh-ins provides an awareness that can help you maintain your weight loss achievement. By keeping you actively involved in maintaining your losses, it empowers you to continue to be successful.

Flex your power

Once you've reached your weight-loss goal on my No Flour, No Sugar Diet, you should feel free to relax the rules a bit. Now that you have mastered the tools for achieving and maintaining your goal weight, you can allow yourself to indulge now and then, confident in the knowledge that you can manage your weight on an ongoing basis. Perhaps you'll want to begin by reintroducing foods that contain flour—an occasional pasta dish or sandwich, for instance—while continuing to avoid foods containing sugar. Don't go crazy, but rather reintroduce these foods slowly and in moderation. And, most important, weigh yourself once a week. If your weight remains constant, continue with your modified version of the diet. You may even allow yourself to indulge in a sugary treat now and then. If, on the other hand, you see the needle on the scale beginning to creep back up, revert to the more restrictive version of the diet. Remember, it's far easier to lose two or three pounds than it is to lose twenty or thirty.

I have received literally hundreds of letters from readers who have successfully tried my No Flour, No Sugar Diet, lost weight, and acknowledged that they are able to stick with the diet indefinitely—using the more restrictive version until they reach their goal weight and then modifying it to suit their ongoing personal needs.

Part III

Getting Down to Business: Your New Eating Plan

Dear Dr. Gott, When my 6-foot-4-inch tall, 39-year-old son weighed 360 pounds, he was found to have high blood pressure, ankle swelling, and a slightly elevated blood sugar level. Obviously something had to be done, but he was reluctant to lose weight and to follow a regular exercise plan—until one of his leg veins burst. He couldn't stop the bleeding and ended up in the emergency room. The experience scared him enough to commit to your No Flour, No Sugar Diet.

In less than a year, he lost 150 pounds. The effects were astounding. His blood pressure and sugar levels are now normal, his legs are slender, and his self-esteem has risen astronomically. This accomplishment has made an enormous difference in his outlook and health. He is justifiably proud of himself and, we, his family, are proud of him as well. I cannot thank you enough for the positive changes you made in virtually saving my son's life. Your diet is simple, inexpensive, and effective. Keep up the good work.

Now that you've got an arsenal of tools to help you adopt new habits that will lead you to your weight loss goals and a lifetime of good health, let's get down to the nitty gritty. In this section, you'll learn how to develop your own eating plan based on the principles of my No Flour, No Sugar Diet and to adapt the diet to suit your particular needs, as well as your likes and dislikes. As you learned in the last section, creating a well thought-out plan—one that you can stick to week in and week out—is crucial to dieting success.

16

What to Eat/What not to Eat

You've already learned that to lose weight successfully on my No Flour, No Sugar Diet, you need to avoid any foods containing flour or added sugar. As a sort of refresher course, here is the list of foods you should avoid and then a list of foods you may enjoy.

Fortunately, the list of foods you can eat is much longer than the list of foods you can't eat.

Foods containing flour and/or sugar to avoid

All-purpose flour	Cakes
Pastry flour	Cookies
Cake flour	Candy
Whole wheat flour	Sodas (non-diet)
Unbleached flour	Ice cream
Rye flour	Pasta
Rice flour	Tortilla chips
Brown rice flour	Crackers
Corn flour	Jam
Bread	Jelly
Bagels	Teriyaki sauce
Croissants	Hoisin sauce
Donuts	Many salad dressings

As you can see by the list below—only a partial list—the foods you are allowed are numerous, varied, healthful, and delicious.

Foods to enjoy

Starches and grains

Rice (white, brown, risotto, wild, etc.)

Oats

Barley

Bulgur

Quinoa

Potatoes

Sweet potatoes and yams

Corn and corn meal (including polenta)

Arrowroot powder

Vegetables and legumes

Beans (garbanzo, soy, kidney, black, white, etc.)

Avocados

Lettuce

Kale

Chard

Spinach

Cabbage

Squash (acorn, butternut, pumpkin, zucchini, etc.)

Tomatoes

Cauliflower

Broccoli

Brussels sprouts

Carrots

Celery

Endive

Radishes

Bell peppers

Green beans

Peas (English peas, snow peas, sugar snap peas)

Nuts and seeds

Almonds

Pistachios

Walnuts

Pecans

Cashews

Pumpkin seeds

Sunflower seeds

Sesame seeds

Soy nuts

Peanut butter and other nut butters (no-sugar-added)

Tahini (sesame paste)

Fruits

Apples

Pears

Berries

Melons

Peaches

Nectarines

Figs

Cherries

Apricots

Grapes

Bananas

Papayas

Mangoes

Pineapple

Dried fruits

Fruit preserves (no-sugar-added)

Meat, Poultry, and Seafood

Fish (especially fatty fishes like salmon and mackerel)

Shellfish (shrimp, scallops, crab, oysters, mussels, etc.)

Chicken

Turkey

Pork tenderloin

Pork chops with visible fat removed

Extra lean ground beef

Lean cuts of beef such as London Broil

Dairy

Eggs (including whole eggs, egg whites, and liquid egg substitutes)

Low-fat, nonfat yogurt (sugar-free; frozen or otherwise)

Low-fat or nonfat milk

Low-fat or nonfat cheese

Cooking fats

Olive oil

Canola oil

Sunflower oil

Safflower oil

Sweets and Treats

No-calorie artificial sweeteners (Splenda, Nutrasweet, etc.)

Fruit sweeteners

Stevia

Sugar-free ice cream (low-fat versions)

Sugar-free frozen yogurt (low-fat versions)

Sugar-free pudding (low-fat versions)

Diet sodas

A word about alcohol

One's favorite alcohol may be consumed in moderation with this diet, but be aware that all alcohol provides empty calories. Wine, especially red wine, has been in the news lately due to its recently discovered beneficial health effects when consumed in moderation.

17

Satisfying Your Sweet Tooth without Sugar

A raging sweet tooth is a weakness shared by many of us. In fact, even newborn infants have been shown to react positively to sweet flavors. And there is historical evidence that this is no modern phenomenon. A 20,000-year-old cave painting shows a Neolithic man snatching honey from a wild bees' nest. It seems that we humans always have always enjoyed our sweet treats. If you're typical, you've likely indulged your sweet tooth regularly throughout your life, which is a hard habit to break. It's so tempting to have something sweet after meals—or just to break up the day. But fear not, there are many ways that you can satisfy your sweet tooth and still stick to the No Flour, No Sugar Diet.

Choose naturally sweet foods

> **Dear Dr. Gott,** *I love your No Flour, No Sugar Diet, but I have a question about the sugar. Are you referring to "sugar added" only? Does the prohibition include foods with natural sweeteners, such as dairy products and fruit?*

> **Dear Reader,** *If the label mentions glucose, sucrose, corn syrup (artificial sweetener), or "sugar added," avoid the product. Natural fruit sugar (fructose) and milk sugar (lactose) are acceptable. The purpose of the diet is to reduce unnecessary calories. Thus, table sugar (cane sugar), which is commonly added to processed foods, is best avoided.*

Ripe, fresh fruits are the ideal way to feed your sweet tooth. Fruit is not only naturally sweet and relatively low calorie, but is also nutrient dense. A medium apple, for instance, is only about ninety calories and is full of vitamins and fiber. Choose fresh seasonal fruits: melons and grapes in the springtime; berries, peaches, nectarines, figs, cherries, apricots, and plums in the summertime; apples and pears in the fall; citrus fruits in the winter. If fresh fruits are hard to find year-round in your area, opt for canned or jarred fruits that are packed in their own juices without added sugar. Fruit preserves are also a satisfying sweet treat. Just be sure to choose fruit-only varieties that do not have sugar added. Dried fruits, too, are a good snack, but keep in mind that having had their water content removed, small amounts can pack a lot of calories. Check the serving size on the label and stick to it.

While added sugar should be avoided, there are many acceptable sugar substitutes available to satisfy you when you just can't fend off your craving for sweets.

Dear Dr. Gott, I am trying hard to follow your No Flour, No Sugar Diet, and I have had great success with it. However, I really need to have a sweetener, such as honey or sugar, in my four cups of coffee a day. I know I should avoid sugar, but is the honey acceptable? Do I have other options?

Dear Reader, The sugar restriction in my diet includes obvious concentrated sweets, including honey, molasses, cane sugar, maple syrup, and corn syrup (a commercial sweetener). Other natural sugars, such as fructose and sucrose, in fresh fruits and vegetables are permitted.

In order to reduce your consumption of calorie-rich sugar products, I suggest that you avoid honey in your coffee and substitute Splenda, a calorie-free sweetening agent derived from sugar that should make your coffee more palatable without adding unnecessary calories.

Try natural sugar substitutes

Since natural sweeteners come from fruits and grains, they have the benefit of containing lots of vitamins and nutrients. They also don't have the unpleasant aftertastes often associated with artificial sweeteners. Unlike artificial sweeteners, they do contain calories, though, so they should be used sparingly.

Fruit sweeteners

Liquid fruit sweeteners, which are made from concentrated fruit juices, are a good substitute for sugar and honey in cooking. These syrups are sweeter than sugar and have fewer calories per serving. In the recipe section of this book, I've included several recipes that use fruit sweeteners, but feel free to experiment on your own. Just remember that since they are sweeter than sugar, you'll need less. Also, since they are in liquid form, you may need to adjust the amount of other liquids in your recipes to accommodate them. They can be found in the baking-needs aisle of health food stores and many supermarkets. (I like the Wax Orchard brand product called Fruit Sweet.)

You can also make your own fruit sweetener by boiling down frozen fruit juice concentrate. Bring the concentrate to a boil in a small saucepan, reduce heat, and simmer until it has thickened a bit, about ten minutes. Apple juice is your best bet, as its mild flavor won't overpower your recipe as other juices might.

Fruit sweeteners do have calories, unlike some of the artificial sweeteners available, so you should still enjoy them only in moderation while on my No Flour, No Sugar Diet.

Agave cactus nectar

This sweetener is made from the core of the agave cactus (the same cactus that is used to make tequila). Like other fruit sweeteners, it is sweeter than sugar, so you'll use less and get fewer calories per serving. Again, this sweetener is a great alternative to sugar in cooking but should be enjoyed only in moderation as it still contains calories.

Stevia

Stevia is an herb that is indigenous to Paraguay and Brazil, where it has been used for centuries as a sweetener for coffee, tea, and food. It has also been used since the 1970s in Japan as a sweetener in everything from sweet soy sauce to Diet Coke. Stevia is a natural, unadulterated, relatively inexpensive food that has been safely consumed for hundreds of years. It has been found to be safe by numerous governments.

It is surprising that stevia has not received more attention as a sugar alternative in this country. After its approval for use in Japan and other Asian countries, it has only been approved for sale in the United States as a "dietary supplement" and cannot be labeled as a sweetener.

Nonetheless, stevia is a wonderful, natural, calorie-free alternative to sugar. You can find it in the herb or dietary supplement sections of most health food stores in either powder or extract form. It can be used as a tabletop sweetener or in cooking. The trouble with using stevia in cooking, however, is that it is many times sweeter than sugar, so it can be difficult to substitute without changing the character of the recipe. One cup of sugar is equal to one teaspoon of stevia powder. One way to make stevia more easily usable in place of sugar in recipes is to dissolve one teaspoon of stevia powder in one cup of water, but you may need to adjust the amount of other liquids in your recipe to make up for the extra water.

There are numerous other natural sweeteners available, but most are too high in calories to be acceptable sugar substitutes. Maple syrup, honey, and molasses, for example, are natural and essentially unprocessed sweeteners, but they pack more calories per serving than regular table sugar, making them unacceptable as substitutes. Likewise, seemingly healthful choices like brown rice syrup and amazake (made from rice and other ingredients) are also higher in calories per serving than is regular table sugar, so they should not be substituted either.

Experiment with no-calorie artificial sweeteners

Artificial sweeteners are a real boon to dieters eager for a way to add sweetness to the foods they eat without adding calories. Unfortunately most of them taste, well, artificial, making them poorly suited for use in large quantities, such as for baking or making desserts. But as tabletop sweeteners—for adding to your coffee or tea or sprinkling over oatmeal, for instance—they're a great way to satisfy your cravings for sweet flavors without the empty calories of sugar.

Saccharin (Sweet 'N Low)

The world's first low-calorie artificial sweetener, saccharin, was discovered in 1879 by researchers at Johns Hopkins University. While there has been controversy over the years regarding the safety of saccharin, it is currently one of the world's most studied foods, and the evidence indicates that it is safe for human consumption. Saccharin is 300 to 500 times sweeter than sugar, so a little goes a long way. Commercial brands of saccharin-based sweeteners (such as Sweet 'N Low) use dextrose, a natural carbohydrate, to dilute it and make it suitable for use as a food additive.

Aspartame (Nutrasweet or Equal)

Aspartame is composed of the amino acids aspartic acid and phenylalanine, which are components found naturally in meats, grains, dairy products, and fruits. The majority of the scientific studies that have been done on aspartame have shown the product to be safe for human consumption. Aspartame is fine to use as a sweetener for coffee or in other ways as a tabletop sweetener. However, when it is heated, as in baking, aspartame has a tendency to lose its sweetness, making it unsuitable as a sugar substitute for cooking.

Dear Dr. Gott, Is it true that consuming diet drinks with aspartame will slow down my metabolism?

Dear Reader, Sugar substitutes such as aspartame do not affect metabolism—except that by taking the place of high-calorie sugar, they force the body to burn unwanted fat for energy. Avoidance of sugar is the cornerstone of any diet program for weight reduction.

Sucralose (Splenda)

Sucralose is a no-calorie sweetener that is made from sugar. To convert regular sugar to sucralose, three chlorine atoms are selectively substituted for three hydrogen-oxygen groups on the sugar molecule. Sucralose is highly stable under a wide range of processing conditions, so it can be used as a substitute for sugar in cooking and baking and as a tabletop sweetener. Because it is made from sugar, its manufacturers claim that it tastes like sugar.

While its flavor is decidedly more natural and "sugar-like" than some other artificial sweeteners, you may notice an unpleasant aftertaste if you use it in large quantities. I prefer to limit its use to tabletop sweetening, as I find the aftertaste unpalatable when it is used as a sweetener in cooking. You should feel free to experiment on your own, however. Sucralose is about 600 times sweeter than sugar, but the Splenda brand product available in supermarkets has other ingredients added so that it measures and sweetens, cup for cup, just like sugar.

Sucralose is relatively new on the artificial-sweetener scene, and there is some skepticism about whether or not it is safe. Although some argue that not enough study has been done on sucralose to justify it, the compound has been approved for use as a sweetener by the FDA and is considered safe.

Dear Dr. Gott, I have had amazing success with your No Flour, No Sugar Diet. It is the easiest plan I have ever tried. I have lost 50 pounds in the last year. I have some questions about substitutions. I have become an avid label reader and I am amazed at the products that contain sugar. Things like nondairy creamer and salad dressings surprised me when I found out some show sugar as the biggest ingredient. It seems there is no cold cereal that does not contain sugar and white flour. Is whole-grain hot cereal acceptable? Are sugar-free ice cream and candy bars allowed?

Dear Reader, I am delighted at your success.

Artificially sweetened products are permitted under my diet; it's the sugar itself that provides the "empty" calories that are anathema to weight control. Whole grain hot cereal is okay, as are unsweetened breakfast cereals that do not list the word "flour" on the package label.

Foods containing sugar alcohols (maltitol, lactitol, sorbitol)

With the booming industry of low-carb foods we've seen in recent years, you may have noticed a lot of new sugar-free or reduced-sugar products appearing on your supermarket's shelves. Many of these products contain sugar alcohols, the most popular of which are maltitol, lactitol, and sorbitol.

Sugar alcohols is a confusing name for these substances, as they are neither sugar nor alcohol. In fact, they are carbohydrates that resemble both sugar and alcohol and are used to add sweetness, as well as bulk and texture, to foods. These compounds, which occur naturally in some foods, are used as sweetening agents in many sugar-free food products, such as candy bars and cookies. At this time, they are not available for use in home kitchens. They have, however, become quite popular in recent years as the public's appetite for sweet-tasting foods that are low in carbohydrates has grown.

Sugar alcohols provide a clean, sugar-like flavor but with significantly fewer calories than sugar. Their calorie content ranges from one and a half to three calories per gram, compared to four calories per gram for sucrose or other sugars. Since they are not calorie-free like sucralose and aspartame, they should be enjoyed in moderation as part of your regular diet. As a general rule of thumb, products containing five grams (or fewer) of sugar alcohols per serving are acceptable on my No Flour, No Sugar Diet. If the food contains more than five grams, however, you have to assume that the sugar alcohol is contributing excess empty calories.

While sugar alcohols occur naturally in many foods, such as fruits and vegetables, and are considered safe for consumption, there are some negative effects. When consumed in excessive amounts, they may cause bloating, diarrhea, or a laxative effect.

18

Satisfying Your Carbohydrate Cravings without Flour

Dear Dr. Gott, I have successfully tried your No Flour, No Sugar Diet, but I have a question. I am a regular runner. What do I eat in place of carbohydrates? I currently consume ground whole wheat bread (no "flour" on the label), whole wheat pasta, brown rice, and potatoes.

Dear Reader, Although I am somewhat surprised that your whole wheat bread and pasta contain no flour, I'll respect your observation that the word "flour" does not appear on their labels. Ordinarily my diet excludes bread and pasta; however, my rule is that if the words "flour," "sugar," or "corn syrup" (commercial sweetener) do not appear on the label, the food is okay to consume. Under the usual circumstances, people can obtain enough carbohydrates from alternative foods; rice, for example, is a good source.

While carbohydrate cravings may be just as strong as sugar cravings for many people, the "no flour" requirement of my No Flour, No Sugar Diet is much easier to satisfy than the no sugar requirement. That is because all carbohydrates are allowed on the diet except for those foods that contain flour. This means that you can still enjoy rice, potatoes, barley, oats, peas, corn, beans, vegetables, and fruits.

You may need to read labels carefully when you first begin the diet so that you can get a sense of which foods contain flour and which don't. For example, many brands of corn tortillas are made with corn flour, while others use only ground corn or corn meal and are perfectly acceptable on the diet. Likewise, tortilla chips usually contain corn flour, although some brands use only corn meal.

If you're craving pasta—or if you find yourself in an Italian restaurant—you might try the risotto (Italian-style rice) instead. If nothing but a sandwich will do, try using bread made from sprouted whole grains—health food stores and many supermarkets carry flour-free breads that are made from sprouted wheat berries, sprouted rye, or sprouted barley. The texture is a bit different from the fluffy flour-based breads you may be used to, but they make a decent sandwich nonetheless. Read labels carefully and watch out for the word "flour." It's the red flag that lets you know the food is not to be consumed while adhering to my No Flour, No Sugar Diet.

As far as side dishes go, there are plenty of starchy alternatives to pasta and bread to go along with your meals. Beans and corn are starchy vegetables that fill you up while providing loads of nutrition and healthful fiber. Tomato sauce-topped polenta—an Italian-style cornmeal mush—is a satisfying alternative to spaghetti marinara. Brown rice, bulgur, and quinoa, too, make hearty side dishes.

Recipes that call for bread crumbs to provide bulk—such as meatloaf or crab cakes—can often be altered successfully by substituting rice, oats, or barley. Recipes that use bread crumbs as a breading on the outside of meats or vegetables that will be fried or baked can be altered by substituting nut meal, which is made from finely ground almonds or hazelnuts.

Dear Dr. Gott, I have been on your No Flour, No Sugar Diet for about a month with great success; I have consistently lost about two pounds a week and find the diet easy to follow. In fact, I have also cut out carrots, potatoes, rice, peas, and lima beans.

My neighbor, a nurse, warns me that because my consumption of fats and proteins is proportionately greater because of the elimination of most carbohydrates, I am in danger of liver and kidney damage. In your opinion, should I be concerned?

Dear Reader, I do not believe that you need to be concerned, one reason being that you are actually consuming less fat (no toast with butter, no pasta with cheese).

However, my diet allows vegetables, so you might consider including them in your daily meals. Let's keep it simple: If a product contains flour or sugar according to the label on the container (or by common sense), avoid it. Thus your diet will primarily be composed of meat, poultry, fish, salads, vegetables, and fresh fruit—a balanced intake without excess calories. This type of broad diet should not lead to organ damage or adverse health consequences. Moreover, the No Flour, No Sugar Diet is not permanent. As I have repeatedly advised, once a person has reached a weight reduction goal, he or she can relax the restrictions and continue to monitor body weight.

Far from leading to health concerns, my diet actually promotes good health by reducing the risk of cardiovascular disease. And, as you've discovered, it's easy and cheap.

One cautionary note about substitutions, however, should be made. Be careful to watch your portion sizes of these foods. Just because a food is allowed on the diet doesn't mean it's a free-for-all. Remember, a calorie is a calorie, so substituting too much of one high-calorie food with too much of another high-calorie food will hardly help you to achieve your weight loss goals.

19

The Meal Plans

On the following pages are two week's worth of simple daily meal plans to get you started on the right foot.

You may want to photocopy these meal plans so you can mark them up to suit your own tastes or individual needs. For instance, if you don't like fish, you may want to cross the fish dishes off the plan and replace them with other dishes—just be careful not to replace a low-calorie meal with a diet-busting feast.

Repeat these fourteen plans exactly as they are for the following two weeks or modify them to fit your individual tastes.

Once you've reached your goal weight, you should feel free to begin experimenting with the reintroduction of foods containing flour or sugar. If you've really been missing pasta, try having it once or twice a week, for example.

Simple Daily Meal Plans

Day 1

Breakfast: Omelet Muffin (p. 112), sliced fresh strawberries
Snack: Diced cantaloupe
Lunch: Greek Salad (p. 122)
Snack: No-sugar-added yogurt
Dinner: Chicken Breasts in Rosemary-Dijon Sauce (p. 147), Spinach Salad with Tomato Vinaigrette (p. 127), steamed brown rice

Day 2

Breakfast: Coconut-Pecan Granola (p. 118), nonfat milk, banana
Snack: Apple with reduced fat cheese
Lunch: Mushroom Soup with Barley (p. 119)
Snack: Eggplant and Tomato Spread (p. 137) with raw vegetables for dipping
Dinner: Roasted Garlic Salmon (p. 142), green salad with vinaigrette dressing, quinoa

Day 3

Breakfast: Whole grain cereal (with no flour or added sugar), nonfat milk, fresh peach
Snack: Diced pineapple
Lunch: Green salad with water-packed tuna, sliced tomato, shredded carrot, and no-sugar-added balsamic vinaigrette
Snack: Spiced Edamame (p. 134)
Dinner: Meatballs in Tomato Sauce (p. 152) and Baked Polenta with Fresh Corn (p. 172)

Day 4

Breakfast: Baked Eggs with Canadian Bacon, Tomatoes, and Feta Cheese (p. 115)
Snack: Apple with no-sugar-added peanut butter
Lunch: Radicchio Salad with Pears, Blue Cheese, and Toasted Pecans (p. 126), grilled or roasted chicken breast

Snack: Spiced Pumpkin Dip (p. 138) with sliced red bell pepper for dipping

Dinner: Broiled Portobello Mushroom "Steaks" with Rosemary Red Wine Reduction (p. 164), oven-roasted potatoes, green salad with balsamic vinaigrette

Day 5

Breakfast: Hearty Four-Grain Cereal (p. 109), banana, nonfat milk

Snack: 1 hard-boiled egg

Lunch: Vietnamese Shrimp Wraps (p. 131)

Snack: Chili-Lime Roasted Chickpeas and Pistachios (p. 134)

Dinner: Seared Pork Chops with Cherry-Balsamic Reduction (p. 157), Stir Fried Sugar Snap Peas with Garlic (p. 168), small baked yam

Day 6

Breakfast: 1 basic Crepe (p. 111) filled with sliced lean ham and reduced-fat cheese; sliced apple

Snack: 1 stalk celery filled with reduced-fat, no-sugar-added peanut butter

Lunch: Taco Salad with Spiced Prawns (p. 124)

Snack: Spiced Edamame (p. 134)

Dinner: Curry Yogurt Chicken (p. 149), steamed or sauteed zucchini, steamed brown rice

Day 7

Breakfast: Feta Cheese Omelet with Zucchini, Peas, and Mint (p. 113)

Snack: 1 part-skim mozzarella cheese stick

Lunch: Green salad with sliced cucumber, tomato, red onion, grilled chicken or water-packed tuna, and balsamic vinaigrette

Snack: Hummus with fresh vegetables

Dinner: Seared Salmon Fillets with Sorrel-Tomato Compote (p. 143), quinoa, oven-roasted asparagus

Day 8

Breakfast: Oatmeal Pancakes (p. 110) with sliced fresh peaches
Snack: 1 stalk celery filled with Laughing Cow Light Cheese or other reduced-fat cheese
Lunch: Cobb Salad Wrap with Balsamic Vinaigrette (p. 129)
Snack: Baked Tortilla Chips (p. 135) with Summer Salsa (p. 135)
Dinner: Curried Lentils with Butternut Squash (p. 160), steamed rice

Day 9

Breakfast: Coconut-Pecan Granola (p. 108), nonfat milk, banana
Snack: Diced melon
Lunch: Fusion Gazpacho with Seafood (p. 118)
Snack: Chili-Lime Roasted Chickpeas and Pistachios (p. 134)
Dinner: Grilled Chicken Strips with Cilantro-Lime Pesto (p. 151), Roasted Brussels Sprouts with Pine Nuts and Parmesan Cheese (p. 168)

Day 10

Breakfast: Frittata with Tender Greens and Fontina Cheese (p. 114)
Snack: 1 stick part-skim mozzarella cheese
Lunch: Green Chili and Cheese Quesadillas (p. 130)
Snack: Sliced roasted turkey breast with reduced-fat cheese
Dinner: Roast chicken, Roasted Winter Vegetables (p. 169), Wild Mushroom and Bulgur Stuffing (p. 172)

Day 11

Breakfast: Hearty Four-Grain Cereal (p. 109)
Snack: Apple with reduced-fat, no-sugar-added peanut butter
Lunch: Green Chili and Cheese Quesadillas (p. 130)
Snack: Baked Tortilla Chips (p. 135) with Zesty Black Bean Dip (p. 136)
Dinner: Stir-Fried Beef with Sugar Snap Peas (p. 154), steamed brown rice

Day 12

Breakfast: 1 Basic Crepe (p. 111) filled with sliced lean ham and re-
duced-fat cheese; sliced apple
Snack: Toasted almonds and apricots
Lunch: Chipotle Tomato and Corn Bisque (p. 120)
Snack: Mushrooms Stuffed with Corn and Goat Cheese (p. 138)
Dinner: Seared Ahi Tuna with Wasabi Sauce (p. 144), steamed rice,
steamed broccoli and cauliflower

Day 13

Breakfast: Omelet Muffin (p. 112), sliced strawberries
Snack: Apple with reduced-fat cheese
Lunch: Greek Salad (p. 122)
Snack: Spiced Pumpkin Dip (p. 138) with fresh vegetables
Dinner: Pork Tenderloin Roasted with Fennel, Apples, Potatoes, and
Onions (p. 156), green salad with balsamic vinaigrette

Day 14

Breakfast: Whole grain cereal, nonfat milk, banana
Snack: Hard-boiled egg
Lunch: Fusion Gazpacho with Seafood (p. 118)
Snack: Zesty Black Bean Dip (p. 136) with Baked Tortilla Chips
(p. 135)
Dinner: Moroccan Chicken Stew with Butternut Squash and Qui-
noa. (p. 150), oven-roasted or steamed cauliflower

Part IV

The Recipes

Breakfast

Breakfast is truly the most important meal of the day. Repeated studies have shown that when people eat breakfast, they eat fewer calories over the course of a day than when they don't eat breakfast. The best breakfasts—those that keep you satisfied until lunch—combine protein, carbohydrates, and unsaturated fats.

Breakfast Recipes

- Coconut-Pecan Granola
- Hearty Four-Grain Cereal
- Oatmeal Pancakes
- Basic Crepes
- Omelet Muffins
- Feta Cheese Omelet with Zucchini, Peas, and Mint
- Frittata with Tender Greens and Fontina Cheese
- Baked Eggs with Canadian Bacon, Tomatoes and Feta Cheese

Coconut Pecan Granola

Less sweet than you may be used to, this granola adds a delicious crunch to yogurt—try it with nonfat plain yogurt with sliced fresh peaches or strawberries. It also makes a delightful topping for fruit crisp and is a perfect quick breakfast on its own with skim milk. Add raisins or other dried fruit for variation.

¾ cup Fruit Sweet
2 tablespoons butter
6 cups old-fashioned oats
¾ cup toasted pecans
¾ cup unsweetened shredded coconut
1 tablespoon vanilla extract
pinch of salt

Preheat oven to 325° F.

Melt butter in a large mixing bowl in the microwave. Add Fruit Sweet, oats, pecans, coconut, vanilla extract, and salt. Mix until well combined. Spray a baking sheet with vegetable oil spray and spread mixture out on the pan in an even layer. Bake, stirring several times, about 25 minutes until mixture is light golden brown. Cool completely. Serve at room temperature. Granola can be stored, in an airtight container, for several weeks.

Makes about 8 cups or 16 servings

Hearty Four-Grain Cereal

This hot cereal makes for a good hearty breakfast on a cold winter morning. Serve topped with sliced fresh bananas, if desired.

Nonstick cooking spray
½ cup old-fashioned rolled oats (not quick cooking)
¼ cup brown rice
¼ cup pearl barley
¼ cup bulgur
½ cup raisins
¼ cup fruit sweetener
¼ teaspoon ground cinnamon
pinch of salt
4 cups water

Preheat oven to 375° F.

Spray an 8" x 8" baking dish with nonstick cooking spray. In prepared baking dish, combine oats, rice, barley, bulgur, raisins, fruit sweetener, cinnamon, salt, and water. Stir to combine. Cover with foil and bake in preheated oven, stirring occasionally, about 1½ hours until grains are tender.

This recipe can be doubled and can also be made ahead. Store covered in refrigerator for up to one week and reheat for 2 minutes or so in the microwave.

Serves 4 to 6.

Oatmeal Pancakes

Using oatmeal in place of flour gives these breakfast treats a good dose of fiber. Top them with fresh fruit—try peaches, strawberries, or bananas—and a dollop of plain yogurt.

2 cups old-fashioned oats
2 tablespoons arrowroot powder*
1½ teaspoons baking powder
½ teaspoon baking soda
¼ teaspoon ground cinnamon
Pinch of salt
½ cup liquid egg substitute
1 cup plain low-fat or nonfat yogurt
1 cup nonfat milk
3 tablespoons fruit sweetener
½ teaspoon vanilla extract

In a medium bowl, combine oats, arrowroot powder, baking powder, baking soda, cinnamon, and salt.

In a large bowl, whisk together egg substitute, yogurt, milk, fruit sweetener, and vanilla extract. Slowly whisk dry ingredients into egg mixture to combine. Let mixture stand 20 to 30 minutes.

Spray a heavy nonstick skillet with canola oil spray or nonstick cooking spray and heat over medium heat. Pour batter, ¼ cup at a time, into skillet and cook until bubbles form on the top of the pancake, about 2 minutes, then flip over and cook until the bottoms begin to brown and pancake is cooked through, about 2 minutes more.

Serves 4.

*Arrowroot powder is a ground starch that can be found in health food stores and many supermarkets

Basic Crepes

Crepes are surprisingly easy to make. The trick is to make sure the batter coats the bottom of the pan evenly and that your heat isn't too high. These light wraps can be used to bundle up anything from ham and cheese to peaches and yogurt to sautéed mushrooms. Experiment with different fillings and try them for breakfast, lunch, dinner, or dessert.

2 large eggs
¾ cup low-fat milk (1%)
6 tablespoons arrowroot powder*
1 teaspoon baking powder
1 tablespoon vegetable oil
¼ teaspoon salt
Vegetable oil spray

In a large bowl, beat eggs with an electric mixer until pale yellow and fluffy, about 2 minutes. Mix in milk, arrowroot, oil, baking powder, and salt.

Spray a nonstick 9- or 10-inch skillet with vegetable oil spray and heat over medium-low heat. Add about 2 tablespoons of the mixture to the hot pan and tilt pan so the mixture is evenly spread over the bottom. Cook until bottom is lightly browned, about 2 minutes, then carefully lift crepe and turn over. Cook until second side is lightly browned, about 2 minutes more. Remove from pan and place between layers of wax paper. Continue until all the batter has been used.

Makes 6 crepes

*Arrowroot powder is a ground starch that can be found in health food stores and many supermarkets

Omelet Muffins

These tasty, flourless "muffins" aren't really muffins at all, but baked scrambled eggs. Try adding leftover vegetables such as sautéed mushrooms, steamed broccoli, or roasted peppers for variation. They're great to have in the refrigerator for hurried weekday mornings. Just pop one in the microwave, and in two minutes you've got a healthful, high protein breakfast. You can even take it with you.

4 large eggs
1½ cups liquid egg substitute
4 ounces diced ham or Canadian bacon
1 cup fresh or frozen corn kernels
3 green onions, thinly sliced
1 teaspoon crumbled dried thyme
3 ounces soft feta cheese, crumbled
1 teaspoon salt
½ teaspoon pepper

Preheat oven to 375° F.

In a large bowl, lightly beat eggs and whisk in egg substitute. Add ham, corn, green onions, thyme, cheese, salt, and pepper, and stir until well combined.

Spray a 12-cup muffin tin with cooking spray. Ladle egg mixture into cups, dividing evenly.

Bake in preheated oven for about 20 to 25 minutes, until tops are puffed and golden and eggs are set. Allow to cool slightly, then run a knife around the edge of the eggs and remove them from the tin. Serve immediately, or cover and refrigerate up to 3 days. To serve, heat on high in microwave for 2 minutes.

Makes 12 servings

Feta Cheese Omelet
with Zucchini, Peas, and Mint

The fresh flavors of spring make this healthy omelet suitable for a fancy brunch, but it's also a perfect casual weekend breakfast.

4 large eggs
1 cup liquid egg substitute
¼ cup water
1 teaspoon salt
½ teaspoon ground pepper
Nonstick cooking spray
½ cup shredded zucchini
¼ cup frozen peas, thawed
¼ cup crumbled feta cheese
¼ cup chopped fresh mint

In a medium bowl, beat together eggs, egg substitute, water, salt, and pepper.

Spray a 10-inch skillet with nonstick cooking spray and heat over medium heat. When pan is hot, add one-fourth of the egg mixture, tilting the pan slightly so that mixture coats the bottom evenly. Cook about 2 minutes, until bottom just begins to set, then place one-fourth each of the zucchini, peas, cheese, and mint down the center of the omelet. Continue to cook until eggs are set, about 3 to 4 minutes more, then fold sides over the vegetables and turn omelet onto a plate. Keep warm while making 4 more omelets in the same manner.

Serves 4.

Frittata with Tender Greens and Fontina Cheese

Frittata is an ideal brunch food—delicious and easy to make for a crowd. It also keeps well, so make up a batch on Sunday and heat up wedges for breakfast during the week.

2 tablespoons olive oil
1 medium shallot, chopped
6 cups baby spinach leaves or arugula
4 large eggs
½ tablespoon arrowroot powder
1 teaspoon salt
½ teaspoon pepper
¼ teaspoon ground nutmeg
4 ounces Fontina cheese, shredded

Preheat broiler.

Heat olive oil in a 10-inch skillet over medium heat. When oil is hot, add shallot and cook, stirring until it becomes soft and translucent, about 3 to 5 minutes. Add greens and cook, stirring, about 2 minutes, until greens are wilted.

In a medium bowl, whisk together eggs, arrowroot powder, salt, pepper, and nutmeg, then pour over greens in skillet and cook, without stirring, until eggs are almost set, about 5 minutes. Sprinkle cheese evenly on top, and place under the preheated broiler for 1 to 2 minutes, until cheese is melted and beginning to brown. Cut into wedges and serve hot.

Serves 4.

Baked Eggs with Canadian Bacon, Tomatoes, and Feta Cheese

These can be made one serving at a time in ramekins or several at a time using a muffin tin.

Per serving:
Olive oil spray or nonstick cooking spray
1 slice Canadian bacon
1 large egg
4 small cherry tomatoes, halved
1 tablespoon crumbled feta cheese
¼ teaspoon crumbled, dried thyme
Salt and pepper

Spray a ramekin or other small, oven-safe dish with olive oil spray or nonstick cooking spray. Place one slice of Canadian bacon in the bottom of the ramekin, top with the egg, then the cherry tomato halves, then the feta cheese. Season with thyme, salt, and pepper. Bake in preheated oven (350°) for 8 to 10 minutes, depending on how many eggs you are cooking at once and how you like them cooked.

Serves 1.

Soups, Salads, and Wraps

If you think sandwiches are the only lunch option, think again. Soups, salads, and wraps provide unending variety for the midday meal.

Soup, Salad, and Wrap Recipes

- Chilled Cucumber Soup with Avocado and Mint
- Fusion Gazpacho with Seafood
- Mushroom Soup with Barley
- Chipotle Tomato and Corn Bisque
- Two-Bean Salad
- Greek Salad
- Black Bean Salad
- Taco Salad with Spiced Prawns
- Radicchio Salad with Pears, Blue Cheese, and Toasted Pecans
- Spinach Salad with Tomato Vinaigrette
- Thai-Style Coleslaw
- Cobb Salad Wrap with Balsamic Vinaigrette
- Green Chile and Cheese Quesadillas
- Vietnamese Shrimp Wraps

Chilled Cucumber Soup
with Avocado and Mint

This beautiful soup makes a sophisticated lunch or starter for a summer evening meal.

3 English cucumbers, roughly chopped (with skin and seeds)
1 large, ripe avocado, diced
1 cup plain low-fat yogurt
1 cup buttermilk
¼ cup balsamic vinegar
Juice of 1 lime
1½ teaspoons salt
12 medium shrimp, peeled and deveined
8 to 10 fresh mint leaves, thinly sliced
4 radishes, slivered

In a large bowl, combine cucumber, avocado, yogurt, buttermilk, vinegar, lime juice, and salt. Transfer in small batches to a blender or food processor. Puree at high speed until smooth.

Strain puree through a fine mesh strainer, cover, and chill until very cold, at least 2 hours. Check seasoning before serving. (Cold soup may need additional salt.)

Just before serving, bring a pot of water to a boil, add the shrimp and 1 tablespoon of salt. Cook until shrimp are pink and cooked through, about 3 minutes. Drain.

Just before serving, place 2 or 3 cooked shrimp in center of each soup bowl. Pour chilled soup over shrimp and garnish with mint and radishes. Serve immediately.

Serves 4 to 6.

Fusion Gazpacho with Seafood

The classic Spanish chilled tomato soup gets spiced up with a hint of jalapeno and a boost of flavor from Asian seasonings. Assorted seafood adds protein while keeping the dish low in fat.

3 15-ounce cans diced tomatoes, with juice
1 to 2 jalapeno chilies, stemmed, seeded, and coarsely chopped
1 medium cucumber, peeled, seeded, and finely diced, divided into 2 parts
1/3 cup fresh basil leaves
1/3 cup fresh mint leaves
1/3 cup fresh cilantro leaves
1 can crab meat, drained and picked over
½ pound bay scallops, blanched in salted water, drained, and chilled
½ pound peeled shrimp, blanched in salted water, drained, and chilled
3 green onions, thinly sliced
½ cup soy sauce
½ cup mirin*
¼ cup olive oil
juice of 2 limes
1 ripe avocado, peeled, pitted, and diced

In a food processor, blend together tomatoes, chilies, half of the diced cucumber, basil, mint, and cilantro until pureed. Pour mixture into a large bowl and stir in lime juice, soy sauce, mirin, olive oil, the remaining diced cucumber, crab meat, scallops, and shrimp. Cover and chill at least one hour and up to 24 hours. Just before serving, stir in diced avocado.

Serves 4 to 6.

*Mirin is a Japanese rice wine that is used for cooking. It can be found in Asian markets or the Asian food aisle of many supermarkets. If Mirin is unavailable, substitute Sake or White Wine.

Mushroom Soup with Barley

This hearty soup is a perfect warm-up on a cold winter night.

1 ounce dried porcini mushrooms
2 cups hot water
2 tablespoons olive oil
3 medium leeks, sliced
2 ribs celery, sliced
1 carrot, peeled and sliced
1 pound fresh mushrooms, sliced
2 teaspoons crumbled dried thyme
2 teaspoons salt
1 teaspoon pepper
½ cup white wine
½ tablespoon arrowroot powder
4 cups beef or vegetable broth
½ cup barley
¼ cup chopped Italian parsley

Cover dried mushrooms with 2 cups hot water. Soak for at least 30 minutes. Strain through a filter, reserving the liquid, and coarsely chop the reconstituted dried mushrooms. Set both reserved mushroom water and chopped mushrooms aside.

In a stockpot, heat the olive oil over medium-high heat until hot, but not smoking. Add the leeks and cook, stirring, until they soften, about 5 minutes. Add celery, carrot, fresh mushrooms, thyme, salt, and pepper and cook, stirring frequently, until the mushrooms soften and begin to brown, about 5 minutes. Stir in wine and cook 1 minute more.

Reduce the heat to medium and add the arrowroot powder and cook, stirring frequently, until thick, about 5 minutes.

Add the broth along with the reserved mushroom water, chopped dried mushrooms, and barley. Return heat to high, and bring to a boil. Reduce heat to medium-low and simmer, covered, for about an hour, stirring occasionally, until the barley is tender and the soup has thickened. Just before serving, stir in parsley. Serve hot.

Serves 6.

Chipotle Tomato and Corn Bisque

Smoky chipotle chilies provide complexity to this rich soup. Using evaporated milk in place of cream keeps it low-fat without sacrificing flavor.

1 tablespoon olive oil
1 medium onion, chopped
2 medium carrots, chopped
2 medium stalks celery, chopped
3 cloves garlic, minced
1 tablespoon chopped fresh oregano or 1 teaspoon dried oregano
1 teaspoon salt
4 cups chicken broth
1 15-ounce can diced tomatoes, with juice
2-4 medium chopped canned chipotle chilies en adobo*, seeds removed
1 15-ounce can corn, drained
1 5-ounce can evaporated milk
Juice of 2 limes
1 medium avocado, diced
½ cup chopped fresh cilantro

Heat olive oil in heavy large pot over medium heat. Add onion, carrot, celery, garlic, and oregano. Cook, stirring frequently, until vegetables soften, about 10 minutes. Add salt, chicken broth, tomatoes with their juice, and chipotles. Raise heat to medium-high and bring mixture to a boil. Reduce heat and simmer, uncovered, about 30 minutes.

Puree soup in a food processor (in batches), or using an immersion blender until smooth. Return soup to pot, stir in corn and evaporated milk, and raise heat again to medium-high. Cook until soup is hot and close to boiling, about 5 minutes. Stir in lime juice. Serve soup topped with chopped cilantro and avocado.

Serves 4 to 6.

*Canned chipotle chilies in adobo sauce ("Chipotles En Adobo") are available at Latin American markets and many supermarkets.

Two-Bean Salad

Middle Eastern spices and raisins give this marinated bean salad an unusual twist. Serve it with Greek Salad (see next page), Eggplant and Tomato Spread (see recipe, p. 137), and purchased stuffed grape leaves for a traditional mezze-style lunch.

1½ tablespoons olive oil
1 medium onion, diced
1 red bell pepper, stemmed, seeded, and diced
1 teaspoon ground cumin
1 teaspoon salt
½ teaspoon ground coriander
½ pound green beans, trimmed
2 14-ounce cans garbanzo beans, rinsed and drained
½ cup raisins
½ cup white wine vinegar

Place green beans in a bowl with 1 tablespoon of water, cover with plastic wrap, and cook in the microwave on high heat about 3 to 5 minutes, until beans are tender. Cut into 1-inch pieces.

Heat the olive oil in a large, heavy skillet over medium high heat. Add onions and cook, stirring, until onions are translucent, about 5 minutes. Add bell pepper and continue to cook, stirring, about 3 minutes. Add cumin, coriander, salt, pepper, garbanzo beans, and raisins. Cook, stirring, another 5 minutes. Transfer mixture to a bowl and add the green beans and wine vinegar. Stir to combine. Let mixture come to room temperature, then cover and refrigerate for at least 24 hours. Bring to room temperature before serving.

Serves 4.

Greek Salad

This quick and simple salad is a perfect accompaniment for grilled chicken or fish.

¼ cup red wine vinegar
1 teaspoon salt
½ teaspoon ground pepper
1 clove garlic, minced
2 tablespoons chopped fresh oregano or 2 teaspoons crumbled dried oregano
1/3 cup olive oil
1 head romaine lettuce, shredded
1 small red onion, diced
1 medium cucumber, peeled, seeded, and diced
3 medium tomatoes, diced
¼ cup pitted Kalamata olives

In a small bowl, mix lemon juice, salt, pepper, garlic, oregano, and olive oil. In a large salad bowl, toss lettuce, onion, cucumber, tomato, and olives. Toss dressing with salad and serve immediately.

Serves 4.

Black Bean Salad

This salad gets better with time. Make it a day ahead and store it, covered, in the refrigerator. Bring to room temperature before serving. To make it a meal, add 2 cups of diced, cooked chicken, shrimp, or smoked tofu.

Juice of 3 limes
1 teaspoon salt
1½ tablespoons fruit sweetener
1 tablespoon ground cumin
1 tablespoon ground coriander
1 tablespoon dried oregano
2 14.5-ounce cans black beans, rinsed and drained
1 can corn, drained
1 cup halved cherry tomatoes
1 medium cucumber, peeled, seeded, and diced
6 green onions, white and light green parts thinly sliced

In a large bowl, combine lime juice, salt, fruit sweetener, cumin, coriander, and oregano. Add beans, corn, tomatoes, cucumber, and onions, and toss until well combined with vinaigrette. If made ahead, cover and refrigerate up to three days. Bring to room temperature before serving.

Serves 4.

Taco Salad with Spiced Prawns

Coating the prawns with spices and broiling them is a quick way to give them lots of flavor without added fat. For the dressing, use mild, medium, or hot salsa depending on your personal taste. I like to use a tangy green tomatillo-based salsa, but red tomato salsa works just as well. Top the salad with a handful of baked tortilla chips for added crunch (just make sure they don't contain flour).

For the prawns:
1 pound medium prawns, peeled and deveined
2 teaspoons mild chili powder
2 teaspoons paprika
½ teaspoon cumin
½ teaspoon oregano
½ teaspoon salt
¼ teaspoon ground chipotle or cayenne (optional)
1 large clove garlic, minced

For the dressing:
½ cup plain low-fat yogurt
½ cup prepared salsa
Juice of one lime

For the salad:
6 cups romaine lettuce, torn into pieces or shredded
1 pint cherry tomatoes, halved
1 medium ripe avocado, peeled and diced
1 cup canned black beans, rinsed and drained

Prepare the prawns:
Preheat broiler.
In a medium bowl, combine chili powder, paprika, cumin, oregano, salt, ground chipotle or cayenne (optional), and garlic. Add prawns and toss to coat evenly with the spice mixture. Spray a baking sheet with nonstick cooking spray or line with foil, and spread prawns out in a single layer. Cook prawns under the broiler, turning once, about 2 minutes per side, until cooked through. Remove prawns from oven and set aside.

Make dressing:

In a small bowl, combine yogurt, salsa, and lime juice. Taste and add salt if desired.

Prepare salad:

In a large salad bowl, toss together lettuce, tomatoes, avocado, and beans. Add dressing, a little at a time, and toss.

Serve salad on individual plates, each topped with several prawns and a scattering of baked tortilla chips, if desired.

Serves 4.

Radicchio Salad with Pears, Blue Cheese, and Toasted Pecans

Bitter radicchio, sweet pears, and salty blue cheese are a match made in heaven. Serve this salad as an elegant first course or alongside grilled chicken or fish.

Juice of 1 large lemon (about ¼ cup)
1 teaspoon Dijon mustard
1½ teaspoons fruit sweetener
½ teaspoon salt
½ teaspoon pepper
¼ to ½ cup olive oil
4 medium heads radicchio, sliced
2 medium, ripe pears cored and sliced into thin wedges
6 ounces crumbled blue cheese
½ cup toasted pecans

In a small bowl, combine lemon juice, mustard, fruit sweetener, salt, and pepper. Whisk in olive oil until well combined.

In a large salad bowl, toss together radicchio, pears, cheese, and vinaigrette. Top with toasted pecans and serve immediately.

Serves 4.

Spinach Salad with Tomato Vinaigrette

Using pureed tomatoes in the vinaigrette cuts down on the amount of fat and calories without compromising on flavor.

1 medium, ripe tomato, seeded and diced
1½ tablespoons red wine or sherry vinegar
½ teaspoon salt
¼ teaspoon ground pepper
¼ cup olive oil
2 tablespoons chopped fresh herbs such as basil, thyme, oregano, rosemary, or cilantro (optional)
6 cups baby spinach leaves
½ medium red onion, diced
2 ounces crumbled feta cheese
2 tablespoons toasted pine nuts

Blend tomatoes, vinegar, salt, and pepper together in a food processor until smooth. Drizzle in olive oil. Stir in herbs, if desired.

In a large bowl, toss together spinach and onion. Add some of the dressing and toss. Add more dressing as needed to lightly coat all of the spinach leaves. Top with crumbled feta and pine nuts and serve immediately.

Serves 4.

Thai-Style Coleslaw

This spicy Southeast Asian slaw is a great match for grilled chicken.

1 small head Napa cabbage, finely shredded
½ small red onion, thinly sliced
1 large carrot, shredded
1 medium cucumber, peeled, seeded and cut into matchstick pieces
¼ cup chopped fresh mint
¼ cup chopped fresh basil
¼ cup chopped fresh cilantro
Juice of 2 limes
2 tablespoons Thai fish sauce or soy sauce
1 teaspoon fruit sweetener
1 serrano or jalapeno chili, seeded and finely chopped

In a small bowl, combine lime juice, fish sauce or soy sauce, fruit sweetener, and chili.

In a large salad bowl, toss together cabbage, onion, carrot, cucumber, mint, basil, and cilantro. Toss with dressing and serve immediately, or cover and refrigerate up to 3 days.

Serves 4.

Cobb Salad Wrap
with Balsamic Vinaigrette

This flavorful wrap will satisfy both your salad cravings and your sandwich cravings at the same time.

¼ cup balsamic vinegar
1 teaspoon Dijon mustard
½ teaspoon salt
½ teaspoon freshly ground pepper
¼ cup olive oil
4 large lettuce leaves
4 slices turkey or chicken breast
Half of a medium, ripe avocado, thinly sliced
12 cherry tomatoes, halved
2 hard-boiled eggs, chopped
2 strips bacon, cooked until crisp, then crumbled
2 ounces crumbled blue cheese

In a small bowl or jar, mix together vinegar, mustard, salt, and pepper. Whisk in oil until well combined.

For each wrap, place one slice of turkey or chicken on top of a lettuce leaf, top with one-fourth of the avocado, 6 cherry tomato halves, one-fourth of the chopped egg, one-fourth of the bacon, and one-fourth of the blue cheese. Drizzle dressing over the filling. Roll up and secure with a toothpick.

Serves 4.

Green Chile and Cheese Quesadillas

Pasilla chilies (also called Poblano chiles) resemble dark, elongated green bell peppers. They're generally only mildly spicy. Feel free to substitute green or red bell peppers if desired. Be sure to use tortillas that are made with corn rather than corn flour.

2 tablespoons olive or vegetable oil
2 cloves garlic, minced
1 medium onion, peeled, halved, and thinly sliced
3 poblano or pasilla chilies, seeded and thinly sliced
¼ cup water
½ teaspoon salt
1 cup Summer Salsa (see recipe, p. 135) or purchased salsa
Olive oil spray or nonstick cooking spray
8 corn tortillas
8 ounces reduced-fat Monterey Jack cheese, shredded

Heat oil in large, heavy skillet over medium-high heat. Add garlic, onions, and chilies. Cook, stirring, until vegetables begin to soften. Add water, cover, and cook, stirring occasionally, until vegetables are soft, about 12 minutes. Remove from heat and stir in salt and salsa.

Spray a large skillet with oil and heat over medium-high heat. Place 1 tortilla in hot skillet, top with one-fourth of the cheese and one-fourth of the vegetable mixture. Top with a second tortilla. Cook until bottom tortilla is golden brown, about 3 minutes. Turn quesadilla over and continue cooking until bottom is golden brown and cheese is melted, about 3 minutes more. Remove from skillet, and cut into wedges. Repeat with remaining tortillas, cheese, and vegetable mixture. Serve immediately.

Serves 4 to 6

Vietnamese Shrimp Wraps

These delicate wraps are perfect for a summer lunch or light dinner on a warm evening. If using crepes as wrappers, make them while the shrimp is marinating, wrap them in aluminum foil, and keep them warm in a 200° oven until ready to serve.

For shrimp:
1½ pounds medium shrimp, peeled and deveined
1 tablespoon minced ginger
1 clove garlic, minced
1/3 cup mirin*
2 teaspoons sesame oil
½ teaspoon salt

For dressing:
Juice of 2 limes
1/3 cup fruit sweetener
3 tablespoons soy sauce
1 large carrot, shredded
2 green onions, thinly sliced
½ teaspoon red pepper flakes

To serve:
1 cup fresh basil leaves
½ cup dry-roasted, lightly salted peanuts, crushed

*Mirin is a Japanese rice wine used for cooking. It is available in specialty markets or in the Asian foods aisles of most supermarkets. If mirin is unavailable, substitute sake or white wine.

Basic Crepes (see recipe, p. 111) or 2 heads butter lettuce or Boston lettuce, leaves removed but kept whole.

In a medium bowl, combine shrimp, ginger, garlic, mirin, sesame oil, and salt. Toss to coat, cover, and refrigerate for 20 to 30 minutes.

In a small bowl, combine lime juice, fruit sweetener, soy sauce, carrot, green onion, and red pepper flakes.

Pour shrimp marinade into a saucepan large enough to hold the shrimp, leaving the shrimp in the bowl. Bring marinade to a boil over medium-high heat. Add shrimp and cook, stirring occasionally, until shrimp are pink and cooked through, 2 to 3 minutes.

Place cooked shrimp on a platter. Arrange lettuce leaves or prepared crepes and basil leaves on the platter. Place crushed peanuts in a small bowl and add that to the platter, along with a small serving spoon. Divide dressing into 4 individual serving bowls, making sure each has some of the shredded carrots and onions. To eat, place 3 shrimp on a lettuce leaf or a crepe, top with 2 or 3 basil leaves, a sprinkle of peanuts, and some of the carrots from the dressing. Roll up and dip into dressing as desired.

Serves 4.

Snacks and Appetizers

It may seem contradictory, but snacking during the day is a great strategy to keep yourself from overeating or bingeing on junk food. By filling up on wholesome, nutritious nibbles at regular intervals, you'll avoid getting so hungry that you're likely to devour everything in sight the minute you get the chance.

Snack and Appetizer Recipes

- Chile-Lime Roasted Chickpeas and Pistachios
- Spiced Edamame
- Baked Tortilla Chips
- Summer Salsa
- Zesty Black Bean Dip
- Eggplant and Tomato Spread
- Spiced Pumpkin Dip
- Mushrooms Stuffed with Corn and Goat Cheese

Chile-Lime Roasted Chickpeas and Pistachios

This is a great healthy snack to have on hand for whenever you crave something salty to munch on.

1 tablespoon paprika
1 tablespoon chili powder
1 teaspoon salt
½ teaspoon cayenne
2 15-ounce cans chickpeas, rinsed and drained
1 cup pistachios
Juice of 1 lime

Preheat oven to 350° F. In a small bowl, mix together paprika, chili powder, salt, and cayenne. Line a baking sheet with aluminum foil, and place chickpeas and pistachios on it. Sprinkle spice mixture over chickpeas and nuts, tossing to coat evenly. Spread chickpeas and nuts out in a single layer and bake in preheated oven, stirring occasionally, until crisp, about 45 to 50 minutes. Squeeze lime juice over mixture, toss, sprinkle with additional salt to taste, and serve immediately—or cool to room temperature and store, in a covered container, for up to 3 days.

Spiced Edamame

These spicy, salty treats are truly addictive. It's a good thing they are high in protein and monounsaturated fat (the "good" fat).

1 pound frozen edamame (soy beans in the pod)
1½ tablespoons coarse sea salt
½ teaspoon paprika
¼ teaspoon (or less) cayenne

Bring a large pot of salted water to a boil. Add edamame and cook 5 minutes. Drain well and transfer to a medium bowl.

In a small bowl, combine sea salt, paprika, and cayenne. Toss salt mixture with edamame. Serve warm or at room temperature.

Serves 4 to 6.

Baked Tortilla Chips

Be sure the tortillas you use for this recipe are made from corn and not corn flour. Use these chips to add crunch to Taco Salad with Spiced Prawns (see recipe, p. 124) or to scoop up Summer Salsa, below, or Zesty Black Bean Dip (next page).

8 corn tortillas, each cut into 8 wedges
Olive oil spray
Salt

Preheat oven to 350° F.

Spread tortilla wedges in a single layer on a baking sheet, and spray lightly with olive oil spray. Bake in preheated oven, turning over halfway through cooking, until lightly browned and crisp, about 15 minutes. Season with salt to taste and serve.

Serves 4.

Summer Salsa

This fresh, spicy salsa is a perfect garnish for tacos, or served as a snack with baked tortilla chips, above.

1 small red onion, chopped
½ teaspoon salt
Juice of 2 limes
4 red or green (or a combination) jalapeno peppers, seeded and finely
    chopped
4 medium tomatoes, chopped
1 cup fresh or frozen (thawed) corn kernels
1 medium, ripe avocado, peeled and diced
1 cup chopped fresh cilantro

Place chopped onion in a bowl, sprinkle with salt, squeeze lime juice over it, and set aside for 15 to 20 minutes. Add chilies, tomatoes, corn, avocado, and cilantro, and stir to combine. Serve immediately— or cover and refrigerate up to 3 days.

Makes about 3½ cups.

Zesty Black Bean Dip

Low in fat and packed with protein and fiber, this festive dip is the perfect party food. Serve it with Baked Tortilla Chips and Summer Salsa (See preceding page.)

1 tablespoon olive oil
2 cloves garlic, minced
½ medium red onion, chopped
1 medium red bell pepper, seeded and diced
2 15-ounce cans black beans, rinsed and drained
Juice of 2 limes
½ cup chopped fresh cilantro
2 teaspoons mild chili powder
1 teaspoon ground coriander
1 teaspoon ground cumin
1 teaspoon salt
½ teaspoon cayenne, or to taste
2 tablespoons water

Heat oil over medium-high heat in a large, heavy skillet. When oil is hot, add garlic, onion, and bell pepper. Cook, stirring until onion is translucent. Remove from heat and set aside.

In a food processor puree beans, lime juice, cilantro, chile powder, cumin, coriander, salt, cayenne, and water, until smooth. Transfer puree to a bowl, and stir in onion mixture. Cover and chill at least 3 hours. Bring to room temperature before serving.

Makes about 2 cups.

Eggplant and Tomato Spread

Serve this chunky Mediterranean-inspired dip with endive fronds for scooping.

2 tablespoons olive oil
1 medium onion, diced
2 cloves garlic, minced
1 large eggplant (about 1½ pounds), peeled and diced
1 teaspoon salt
1 cup diced tomatoes (fresh or canned)
Juice of 1 lemon
¼ cup toasted pine nuts

Heat olive oil in a large heavy skillet over medium-high heat. Add onions and garlic, and cook, stirring occasionally, until onions begin to soften. Add eggplant, salt, and pepper, and cook, stirring until eggplant begins to brown, about 5 minutes. Add tomatoes, cover, and cook about 10 minutes more, until eggplant is tender. Transfer mixture to a bowl, add lemon juice, and mix well. Cool to room temperature. Just before serving, stir in toasted pine nuts.

Serves 4.

Spiced Pumpkin Dip

This easy dip resembles a lighter version of hummus. Serve it with fresh vegetables—endive leaves, celery, carrots, bell peppers—for a light but festive appetizer.

1 15-ounce can pureed pumpkin
2 tablespoons tahini
1 clove garlic, minced
1 teaspoon salt
½ teaspoon ground cumin
¼ teaspoon ground coriander
¼ teaspoon paprika
¼ teaspoon cayenne (optional)
Juice of 1 lemon

In a medium bowl, combine pumpkin, tahini, garlic, salt, cumin, coriander, paprika, cayenne, and lemon juice. Stir until well combined. Serve immediately—or cover and refrigerate for up to 3 days.

Mushrooms Stuffed with Corn and Goat Cheese

These bite-sized morsels are an elegant hors d'oeuvre. Use 4 large portobello mushroom caps in place of the button or cremini mushrooms and serve as a main course. (You may need to broil the mushrooms a bit longer in the first step.)

Olive oil spray
1 pound large button or cremini mushrooms, stems removed and chopped, caps left whole
2 tablespoons olive oil
3 cloves garlic, minced
1 large shallot, minced
½ pound shitake mushrooms, chopped
¼ cup red wine
1 tablespoon chopped fresh thyme

1 tablespoon chopped fresh oregano
1 teaspoon salt
1 teaspoon pepper
1 cup fresh or frozen corn kernels
½ cup low-fat sour cream or crème fraiche
4 ounces crumbled feta cheese

Preheat broiler.

Place whole mushroom caps on a baking sheet with stem side down, spray with olive oil spray, and season with salt and pepper. Broil mushrooms for 3 to 5 minutes, until tender. Pour off any liquid that has accumulated in the pan, and turn mushrooms over so that they are stem side up.

Heat olive oil in large, heavy skillet over medium-high heat. Add garlic and shallots and cook, stirring, until shallots soften, about 3 minutes. Add chopped mushroom stems and chopped shitakes and cook, stirring occasionally, about 5 minutes, until mushrooms have softened and given up their juice. Stir in thyme, oregano, salt, pepper, and wine, and continue to cook, stirring until liquid has evaporated. Add corn and cook 2 minutes more. Lower heat to medium-low, and add sour cream or crème fraiche. Simmer about 2 minutes until cream has begun to be absorbed. Stir in cheese and taste for seasoning.

Spoon filling into mushroom caps, and cook under broiler until tops are lightly browned, about 5 minutes.

Makes about 40 stuffed mushrooms

23

Entrees

Healthful main courses don't need to be difficult or time-consuming to make. This chapter provides recipes for everything from homey casseroles to fancy dishes worthy of company. And best of all, most are quick and easy to prepare, and all will fit easily into your No Flour, No Sugar diet.

Entree Recipes

- Baked Halibut with Fennel, Sun-Dried Tomatoes, and Olives
- Roasted Garlic Salmon
- Seared Salmon Fillets with Sorrel-Tomato Compote
- Seared Ahi Tuna with Wasabi Sauce
- Thai-Style Shrimp in Coconut Milk
- Turkey Sausage, Shrimp, and Brown Rice Jambalaya
- Chicken Breasts in Rosemary-Dijon Sauce
- Pan Roasted Chicken with Bacon, Olives, and Prunes
- Curry Yogurt Chicken
- Moroccan Chicken Stew with Butternut Squash and Quinoa
- Grilled Chicken Strips with Cilantro-Lime Pesto
- Meatballs in Tomato Sauce
- Stir-Fried Beef with Sugar Snap Peas
- Pork Tenderloin Roasted with Fennel, Apples, Potatoes, and Onions
- Seared Pork Chops with Cherry-Balsamic Reduction
- Shepherd's Pie
- Curried Lentils with Butternut Squash
- White Bean Stew
- Eggplant "Lasagne"
- Broiled Portobello Mushroom "Steaks" with Rosemary-Red Wine Reduction
- Broiled Tofu and Vegetables with Peanut Sauce

Baked Halibut with Fennel, Sun-Dried Tomatoes, and Olives

Crisp, juicy, and flavorful fresh fennel bulb keeps the fish moist while it cooks and balances the saltiness of the olives.

Olive oil spray or nonstick cooking spray
2/3 cup pitted Kalamata olives, chopped
¼ cup chopped sun-dried tomatoes in olive oil
2 tablespoons oil from the sun-dried tomatoes
1 large garlic clove, minced
1 bulb fennel, very thinly sliced
4 halibut fillets, about 6 ounces each
¼ cup white wine
2 tablespoons shredded fresh basil

Preheat oven to 400° F.

Mix together olives, sun-dried tomatoes, sun-dried tomato oil, and garlic.

Spray a baking dish large enough to hold the fish in a single layer with olive oil spray or nonstick cooking spray. Place fennel slices in a single layer on the bottom of the dish. Place fish fillets on top of the fennel slices, then top with the olive mixture, dividing it equally among the fillets. Pour the wine over the fish, top with shredded basil, cover the dish with foil, and bake 12 to 15 minutes, until fish is cooked through. Serve immediately.

Serves 4.

Roasted Garlic Salmon

Roasting the garlic brings out its sweetness, which complements the salmon nicely. Serve a spinach salad alongside for a healthy and satisfying meal.

1 medium head garlic, top sliced off so that the tops of the cloves are
    exposed
3 tablespoons olive oil, divided
½ teaspoon salt
½ teaspoon ground pepper
1 tablespoon chopped fresh rosemary or oregano
Juice of 1 lemon
4 6-ounce salmon fillets (each about 1-inch thick)

Preheat oven to 400° F.

Place the garlic on a square of foil. Drizzle 1 tablespoon of the olive oil over the garlic, and wrap up tightly. Roast in oven for about 40 minutes, until garlic is soft.

Squeeze garlic cloves out of the skin and place in a small bowl. Add salt, pepper, and rosemary or oregano, and mash with a fork into a paste. Add remaining 2 tablespoons of olive oil and lemon juice, and stir to combine.

Increase oven temperature to 450° F.

Place salmon on baking sheet, season with salt and pepper, and spread the garlic mixture over the fillets, dividing evenly among them.

Bake salmon uncovered in preheated oven, until cooked through, about 15 to 20 minutes. Serve immediately.

Serves 4.

Seared Salmon Fillets
with Sorrel-Tomato Compote

The spring herb sorrel looks similar to baby spinach, but has a strong tangy flavor to it. Here it provides a bright, fresh note to a simple salmon dish.

1 tablespoon olive oil
4-6 ounce salmon fillets (each about 1-inch thick)
1 tablespoon butter
1 medium shallot, chopped
1 14-ounce can diced tomatoes, drained
1 teaspoon salt
½ teaspoon ground pepper
¼ cup dry white wine
½ cup (packed) chopped fresh sorrel

Season salmon fillets with salt and pepper. Heat olive oil in a large heavy skillet over medium-high heat. When oil is hot, add salmon fillets and cook about 3 minutes per side, until lightly browned. Remove salmon from pan, and set aside.

Add butter to pan. When butter is melted, add shallot, and cook, stirring until shallot begins to soften, about 3 minutes. Add tomatoes to skillet, and cook, stirring about 2 minutes. Add wine and sorrel and cook, stirring about 1 minute more, until sauce is thick and sorrel has wilted. Add seared salmon to pan, reduce heat, and simmer until salmon is hot, about 2 minutes. Serve immediately.

Serves 4.

Seared Ahi Tuna with Wasabi Sauce

This is a great recipe for getting a healthy dinner on the table fast. Serve this with a simple salad of julienned cucumbers, red bell peppers, and carrots with a rice wine vinaigrette.

2 tablespoons wasabi paste*
2 tablespoons water
1/3 cup soy sauce
1 tablespoon vegetable oil
2 tablespoons dry white wine
2 teaspoons sesame oil
1 tablespoon minced fresh ginger
4 green onions, thinly sliced
Canola oil spray or nonstick cooking spray
4 1-inch thick, 6-ounce Ahi tuna steaks
Salt and pepper
2 tablespoons toasted sesame seeds

In a medium bowl, combine wasabi paste, water, soy sauce, vegetable oil, wine, 1 teaspoon of the sesame oil, and ginger. Stir in green onions. Set aside.

Spray a large, heavy skillet generously with canola oil or nonstick cooking spray, add the remaining 1 teaspoon of sesame oil, and heat over high heat. Season tuna with salt and pepper. When pan is very hot, add tuna and sear until browned on the outside but still pink on the inside, about 2 minutes per side. Serve tuna hot with wasabi sauce spooned over the top.

Serves 4.

*Wasabi paste is a Japanese horseradish paste, which can be found in Asian markets or in the Asian foods aisle of many supermarkets. If you can't find wasabi paste, substitute prepared horseradish.

Thai-Style Shrimp in Coconut Milk

This quick shrimp dish is surprisingly satisfying. Serve it over small scoops of steamed brown rice that will soak up the spicy broth.

2 cloves garlic, peeled
1-inch piece of ginger, peeled and diced
2 to 4 jalapeno chilies (to taste), stemmed and seeded
½ cup (packed) fresh cilantro leaves
Juice and zest of 1 lime
1 teaspoon salt
1 14-ounce can light, unsweetened coconut milk
2 tablespoons olive oil
½ cup white wine
2 pounds shrimp, peeled and deveined

In a food processor, combine the garlic, ginger, chilies, cilantro, lime zest, lime juice, salt, and olive oil. Process to a coarse puree.

Place wine and coconut milk in a large pot set over high heat. Stir in cilantro mixture, and bring to a boil. Reduce heat to medium-high, and simmer broth for about 5 minutes. Add shrimp, cover, and cook until shrimp are pink and cooked through, about 4 minutes. Serve shrimp immediately. Ladle into soup bowls along with the broth.

Serves 4.

Turkey Sausage, Shrimp, and Brown Rice Jambalaya

Substituting turkey sausage for the usual high-fat variety and using brown rice in place of white makes this version of the Louisiana classic far healthier.

2 tablespoons olive oil
1 large onion, diced
2 cloves garlic, minced
2 stalks celery, diced
1 green bell pepper, seeded and diced
1 red bell pepper, seeded and diced
¾ pound spicy turkey sausage, thinly sliced
1 tablespoon chili powder
2 teaspoons dried thyme
½ teaspoon cayenne pepper
1 teaspoon salt
1½ cups uncooked brown rice
1 14-ounce can diced tomatoes, drained
6 cups chicken or vegetable broth
¾ pound peeled shrimp

Heat oil in large pot over medium-high heat. Add onion, garlic, celery, and peppers, and cook, stirring until onion is soft and translucent, about 5 minutes. Add sausage, chili powder, thyme, cayenne, and salt. Stir to combine and cook for about 1 minute. Add tomatoes, broth, and rice. Bring mixture to a simmer, reduce heat to low, cover, and cook until rice is tender, stirring occasionally, about 45 minutes. Just before serving, raise heat to high, add shrimp, and cook, stirring, until shrimp is cooked through, about 3 minutes more. Serve hot.

Serves 4 to 6.

Chicken Breasts
in Rosemary-Dijon Sauce

This quick, easy pan sauce gets sophisticated flavors of mustard and wine from the Dijon mustard. Evaporated milk lends creaminess without a lot of added fat and calories.

1 tablespoon olive oil

4 skinless, boneless chicken breast halves, pounded to ¾-inch thickness

½ cup chicken broth

¼ cup Dijon mustard

¼ cup nonfat evaporated milk

1 tablespoon chopped fresh rosemary or 1 teaspoon crumbled dried rosemary

½ teaspoon salt

¼ teaspoon ground pepper

Juice of ½ lemon

4 green onions, white and light green parts only, thinly sliced

Heat olive oil in a large, heavy skillet over medium-high heat. When oil is hot but not smoking, add chicken and cook until nicely browned, about 2 minutes per side. Remove chicken from skillet and set aside. To the skillet, add broth, mustard, evaporated milk, rosemary, salt, and pepper. Bring mixture to a boil and cook, stirring and scraping up any browned bits stuck to the bottom of the pan, about 2 minutes. Return chicken to skillet and simmer until chicken is cooked through and sauce has thickened, about 3 to 4 minutes per side. Add lemon juice and green onions, stir to combine, and serve immediately.

Serves 4.

Pan Roasted Chicken
with Bacon, Olives, and Prunes

This easy baked chicken dish combines salty, sweet, and sour for an unusually sophisticated result. The small amount of bacon seems contraindicated, but it's just enough to add flavor without ruining your diet. Buy your bacon from a butcher so that you can buy only as many strips as you need for your recipe.

2 chicken breasts, split into halves
2 cloves garlic, thinly sliced
1 medium shallot, chopped
1½ tablespoons crumbled dried oregano
1 teaspoon salt
½ teaspoon pepper
¼ cup red wine vinegar
¼ cup olive oil
½ cup dry white wine
2/3 cup pitted prunes, halved
½ cup pitted Spanish green olives
2 strips bacon, diced

Preheat oven to 350° F.

In a large bowl, combine garlic, shallot, oregano, salt, pepper, vinegar, olive oil, and wine.

Arrange chicken pieces in a single layer in a baking dish. Scatter prunes and olives over the chicken and pour marinade over the top. Sprinkle diced bacon over the chicken.

Bake chicken in preheated oven for about 50 minutes, basting occasionally with the pan juices, until chicken is cooked through. Serve immediately.

Serves 4.

Curry Yogurt Chicken

Cooking chicken in yogurt makes it extremely tender and ensures that the flavorful spices really permeate the meat. Steamed brown rice and green beans make perfect accompaniments.

4 skinless, boneless chicken breast halves
2/3 cup plain low-fat or nonfat yogurt
¼ cup light mayonnaise
1 clove garlic, minced
1 tablespoon minced fresh ginger
Juice of one lemon
2 tablespoons curry powder
¼ to ½ teaspoon cayenne (optional)
3 green onions, thinly sliced
1 teaspoon salt

Preheat oven to 375° F.

Place chicken breasts in a baking dish and season with salt and pepper.

In a medium bowl, combine yogurt, mayonnaise, garlic, ginger, lemon juice, curry powder, cayenne (if desired), and green onions. Pour over chicken and turn to coat chicken on all sides.

Bake chicken, uncovered, in preheated oven until cooked through, about 25 minutes.

Serves 4.

Moroccan Chicken Stew
with Butternut Squash and Quinoa

This one-pot meal is packed with protein, fiber, and other important nutrients.

2 tablespoons olive oil
1 pound skinless boneless chicken breast meat, cut into 1-inch pieces
1½ teaspoons salt
1 teaspoon pepper
1 medium red onion, diced
2 cloves garlic, minced
2 tablespoons curry powder
2 teaspoons ground cumin
1 teaspoon ground cinnamon
1 pound butternut squash, peeled and diced
2 14-ounce cans chicken broth
½ cup raisins
1 14-ounce can diced tomatoes, drained
1 cup quinoa
½ cup slivered almonds

Sprinkle salt and pepper over diced chicken. Heat 1 tablespoon of the olive oil in a large, heavy pot over medium-high heat. When oil is hot, add chicken and sauté, stirring frequently until opaque but not cooked through, about 3 minutes. Remove chicken from pan and set aside.

Add remaining tablespoon of olive oil to pot. When oil is hot, add onion and garlic and cook, stirring until onion begins to soften and turn golden, about 4 minutes. Add curry powder, cumin, and cinnamon, and cook another minute or so. Add squash, broth, tomatoes, and raisins. Cover and simmer until squash is tender, about 15 minutes. Add quinoa and continue to simmer, covered, another 15 minutes or until quinoa is tender. Add chicken and simmer uncovered, until chicken is hot and cooked through, about 5 minutes more. Serve immediately, garnished with slivered almonds.

Serves 4 to 6.

Grilled Chicken Strips
with Cilantro-Lime Pesto

Packed with flavor, this quick sauce is all you need to jazz up plain grilled chicken. It's also great on grilled shrimp or broiled tofu.

2 cups packed fresh cilantro leaves
2 cloves garlic
1 or 2 jalapeno chilies, stemmed and seeded
¼ cup dry roasted peanuts, divided
Juice and zest of 1 lime
1 tablespoon Asian fish sauce or soy sauce
1 teaspoon sesame oil
½ teaspoon salt
3 tablespoons olive oil
Vegetable oil spray
1 pound boneless, skinless chicken breast, cut into strips
3 green onions, thinly sliced

In a food processor, puree cilantro, garlic, chilies, half of the peanuts, lime zest and juice, fish sauce or soy sauce, sesame oil, and salt. Add olive oil, and process until smooth, about 1 minute.

Spray chicken strips with vegetable oil spray, and season with salt and pepper. Cook on hot grill or grill pan over medium-high heat, turning once, until cooked through, about 4 minutes per side. Serve chicken over brown rice with pesto drizzled over the top. Garnish with chopped green onions and remaining peanuts.

Serves 4.

Meatballs in Tomato Sauce

Serve these hearty meatballs over Baked Polenta with Fresh Corn (see recipe, p. 172) for a satisfying meal.

For sauce:
1 tablespoon olive oil
1 medium onion, chopped
2 cloves garlic, minced
1 32-ounce can tomato puree or crushed tomatoes
¼ cup dry red wine
1 tablespoon chopped fresh oregano, or 1 teaspoon dried oregano
1 teaspoon salt

For meatballs:
2 large eggs, lightly beaten
½ cup cooked rice (preferably brown rice)
¼ cup finely grated Parmesan cheese
1 tablespoon olive oil
¼ cup chopped fresh Italian parsley
2 cloves garlic, minced
1 teaspoon salt
½ teaspoon pepper
½ pound ground turkey
½ pound ground veal or lean beef

Preheat oven to 450° F.

Heat 1 tablespoon of olive oil in a large, heavy saucepan over medium-high heat. When oil is hot, add onions and garlic, and cook, stirring until onions are soft, about 4 minutes. Add tomato puree, wine, oregano, and salt, and bring to a boil. Lower heat and simmer, uncovered, until thickened, about 30 minutes.

While sauce is simmering, combine eggs, rice, cheese, olive oil, parsley, garlic, salt, and pepper in a large bowl. Add both kinds of ground meat, and mix thoroughly. Form mixture into 1½-inch diameter meatballs.

As balls are prepared, place them on a baking sheet that has been sprayed with olive oil or nonstick cooking spray. When all of the meat mixture has been formed into balls, bake them in the preheated oven for about 20 minutes, until browned and cooked through.

Transfer the cooked meatballs to the tomato sauce, cover the pot and simmer, stirring occasionally, until meatballs are completely cooked through, about 5 minutes more. Serve sprinkled with extra Parmesan cheese, if desired.

Serves 4.

Stir-Fried Beef with Sugar Snap Peas

Quick, flavorful, and healthy—a perfect weeknight dinner. Add a side of steamed brown rice to round out the meal.

2 tablespoons soy sauce
1 teaspoon fruit sweetener
½ teaspoon salt
1¼ pound London Broil, cut across the grain into ¼-inch-thick slices
2 tablespoons cornstarch
2 tablespoons soy sauce
½ cup chicken or beef broth or water
2 tablespoons sherry, mirin*, or white wine
1 tablespoon fruit sweetener
1 tablespoon sesame oil
3 tablespoons vegetable oil
2 tablespoons minced peeled fresh ginger
2 cloves garlic, minced
2 red jalapenos, seeded and minced
2 green jalapeno chiles, seeded and minced
1 medium red bell pepper, seeded and diced
1 pound sugar snap peas, trimmed

In a medium bowl, combine soy sauce, fruit sweetener, and salt. Add the beef, stir to coat, and marinate for 20 to 30 minutes.

While beef is marinating, combine cornstarch, soy sauce, broth, and sherry, mirin, or white wine in a small bowl. Stir until cornstarch has dissolved. Stir in the sesame oil. Set aside.

*Mirin is a Japanese rice wine used for cooking. It is available in specialty food stores and the Asian foods aisle of many supermarkets. If you can't find mirin, substitute Sake or white wine.

Heat 2 tablespoons of the vegetable oil in a large heavy skillet over high heat until hot, but not smoking. Add the beef in batches and cook, stirring until it is no longer pink, about 1 minute per batch. As beef is cooked, transfer it to a plate.

When all the beef is cooked, add the remaining tablespoon of vegetable oil to the pan, and add the ginger, garlic, and jalapenos, and stir fry for 30 seconds. Add the snow peas and bell pepper and cook for another minute. Add 1/3 cup water, cover, and steam the vegetables until they are tender, about 5 minutes. Stir the sauce and add it and the beef to the vegetables, along with any juices that have accumulated. Cook the mixture, stirring, until the sauce thickens and the beef is hot, about 2 minutes more. Serve immediately over steamed brown rice, if desired.

Serves 4.

Pork Tenderloin Roasted with Fennel, Apples, Potatoes, and Onions

Pork tenderloin is very lean and is delicious paired with hearty winter vegetables and apples.

1 large pork tenderloin (about 1 pound)
1 pound new potatoes, halved (quartered, if large)
3 tablespoons olive oil, divided
2 tablespoons whole grain Dijon mustard
1 large onion, sliced
1 medium Granny Smith apple, peeled, cored, and sliced
1 large fennel bulb, sliced
½ cup white wine

Preheat oven to 450° F. Season pork with salt and pepper.

Bring a pot of water to a boil and add potatoes. Boil potatoes about 6 minutes. Drain.

Heat 2 tablespoons of the olive oil in a large, oven-safe skillet over high heat. When the oil is very hot, add pork and sear, turning occasionally, until browned on all sides, about 5 to 7 minutes total. Transfer pork to a plate. Cool slightly. Spread mustard over top and sides of pork.

Add remaining 1 tablespoon of olive oil to the skillet. Add onion, apple, and fennel, and cook, stirring regularly, over medium-high heat until soft and beginning to brown, about 8 minutes. Stir in potatoes, salt, and pepper and spread mixture out evenly in skillet. Place pork on top of vegetable mixture, place skillet in the preheated oven, and roast until vegetables are soft and browned and a meat thermometer inserted into the center of the pork registers 150° F., about 20 minutes. Remove from oven, stir wine into vegetable mixture, cover loosely with foil, and let rest 5 minutes.

Cut pork on the diagonal into ½-inch-thick slices. Spoon apple-onion mixture onto plates. Top with pork and serve.

Serves 4.

Seared Pork Chops with Cherry-Balsamic Reduction

This sauce seems terribly fancy but is surprisingly easy to prepare. The cherries and balsamic lend sweetness that complements the pork nicely. Be sure your chops aren't too thick, though, or you'll end up with tough, dry meat.

4 boneless pork chops (each about ¾-inch thick)
1 tablespoon olive oil
½ medium red onion, diced
¼ cup balsamic vinegar
½ cup dry red wine
¾ cup chicken broth
¾ cup dried cherries (about 1½ ounces)
½ teaspoon salt
¼ teaspoon ground pepper
1 tablespoon chopped fresh rosemary or 1 teaspoon crumbled dried rosemary

Season pork chops with salt and pepper.

In a large, heavy skillet, heat olive oil until very hot. Add pork chops and cook until nicely browned, about 3 minutes per side. Transfer pork to a plate and set aside. Lower heat to medium, and add onion to skillet. Cook, stirring, until onion is soft and translucent, about 3 minutes. Add vinegar, wine, broth, dried cherries, salt, pepper, and rosemary. Bring to a boil, and cook about 5 minutes until sauce begins to thicken. Return pork chops to skillet with sauce and continue to simmer until pork is cooked through, about 3 minutes more per side. Serve chops immediately topped with some of the sauce.

Serves 4.

Shepherd's Pie

This diet-friendly twist on a hearty classic is chock full of vegetables. Substituting pureed cauliflower for half of the potato in the mashed topping lightens up the dish while still giving you the satisfaction of creamy mashed potatoes.

Topping:
1 medium head cauliflower, trimmed and roughly chopped
2 medium potatoes, peeled and diced
¼ cup low-fat sour cream
2 tablespoons butter
1 teaspoon salt
Paprika for garnish

Meat filling:
2 tablespoons olive oil
1 medium onion, diced
½ pound mushrooms, chopped
2 medium carrots, peeled and diced
1¼ lb. extra lean ground beef
1 teaspoon salt
½ teaspoon pepper
1 teaspoon crumbled dried thyme
1 cup fresh or frozen peas
1 tablespoon tomato paste

Preheat oven to 375° F.

Bring a large pot of water to a boil, and add diced potatoes. Cook until potatoes are tender, about 15 minutes. Drain.

While potatoes are cooking, place chopped cauliflower in a large bowl with 2 tablespoons of water. Cover with plastic wrap and microwave on high, 10 to 12 minutes, until cauliflower is tender. Transfer cauliflower to a food processor and process to a smooth puree.

Place cooked potatoes in a large bowl and mash until smooth. Mix in butter, sour cream, salt, and pureed cauliflower. Set aside.

Heat 1 tablespoon of the olive oil in a large, heavy skillet over medium-high heat. When oil is hot, add onion and carrot and sauté until onion is translucent. Add mushrooms, and cook, stirring until mushrooms are soft and liquid has evaporated, about 5 minutes more. Remove mushroom mixture from pan and set aside.

Without washing pan, add remaining 1 tablespoon of olive oil, and heat over medium-high heat until hot. Add ground beef and cook, stirring and breaking up meat, until browned, about 5 minutes. Stir in salt, pepper, thyme, peas, and tomato paste. Mix meat mixture into onion, carrot, and mushroom mixture.

Spray a 9-inch x 13-inch baking dish with olive oil spray or nonstick cooking spray. Fill dish with meat mixture and spread into an even layer. Top with mashed potato-cauliflower topping and spread into an even layer. Sprinkle paprika over the top, and bake in preheated oven about 45 to 50 minutes, until lightly browned on top. Serve hot.

Serves 6 to 8.

Curried Lentils with Butternut Squash

Using pre-chopped squash saves a lot of time. If you can't find pre-cut squash, try piercing the whole squash several times with a sharp knife, then microwaving it on high for 1 to 2 minutes. This will soften the squash and make it much easier to peel.

3 cups peeled butternut squash in ½-inch pieces (about 1 pound)
1 small onion, diced
Olive oil spray
1 tablespoon curry powder
½ teaspoon salt
¼ teaspoon pepper
¼ teaspoon cayenne or less (optional)
¼ cup chopped pecans
1 cup vegetable broth, chicken broth, or water
2/3 cup lentils
Juice of 1 lime
¼ cup plain low-fat or nonfat yogurt

Preheat oven to 425° F.

Spray a baking sheet with olive oil spray. Toss together squash, onion, curry powder, salt, pepper, and cayenne (optional). Spray mixture all over with olive oil spray, then spread in a single layer on the baking sheet. Bake in a preheated oven for 15 minutes. Stir squash mixture, and spread out again into a single layer. Sprinkle pecans over squash and bake until squash is very tender and pecans are toasted, about 10 minutes more.

While squash is baking, bring broth or water to a boil in a small saucepan. Stir in lentils, reduce heat, and simmer until just tender, about 10 to 15 minutes, depending on the size of your lentils.

In a medium bowl, combine cooked lentils, squash mixture, and lime juice. Toss to combine. Serve hot, topped with dollops of yogurt.

Serves 4 as a side dish.

White Bean Stew

T his hearty vegetarian stew serves as a filling meat-free entree and is also a nice side dish with roasted or grilled chicken.

    2 tablespoons olive oil
    4 cloves garlic, minced
    2 medium shallots, chopped
    ½ pound zucchini, diced
    1 14-ounce can diced tomatoes, drained
    2 14-ounce cans white beans (such as cannellini, great northern
        or navy), rinsed and drained
    1 teaspoon salt
    1 teaspoon pepper
    2 tablespoons chopped fresh oregano
    ½ cup almond meal
    ½ cup grated Parmesan cheese

Preheat oven to 475° F.

Heat oil in 2-quart, oven-safe pot over medium-high heat. Add garlic and shallot, and cook, stirring until onion is soft and translucent, about 5 minutes. Add zucchini, tomatoes, beans, salt, pepper, and oregano, and cook until heated through. Combine almond meal and grated cheese, and sprinkle over the beans. Bake beans in preheated oven until top is golden brown and crisp, about 10 minutes. Serve hot.

Serves 4 as an entree, 6 to 8 as a side dish.

Eggplant Lasagne

This noodle-less lasagne makes for a satisfying flour-free vegetarian entree. Serve it with a green salad with vinaigrette dressing.

Sauce:
1 tablespoon olive oil
1 clove garlic, minced
¼ teaspoon dried hot red-pepper flakes
1 tablespoon chopped fresh rosemary, or 1 teaspoon crumbled dried
    rosemary
2 14-ounce cans diced tomatoes, one with juice, one drained
½ teaspoon salt

Eggplant:
2 medium eggplants, peeled and sliced into 1/8-inch slices
1 tablespoon salt

Filling:
1½ cups part-skim ricotta cheese (about 12 ounces)
½ cup plus 2 tablespoons finely grated Parmigiano-Reggiano cheese
    (about 1½ ounces)
¼ teaspoon black pepper
½ teaspoon salt

Preheat broiler.

Layer eggplant slices, sprinkled with the tablespoon of salt, in a colander which is set in the sink or over a bowl. Let sit 20 to 30 minutes.

In a medium, heavy saucepan, heat olive oil over medium-high heat. Add garlic, and cook, stirring until garlic just begins to color, about 30 seconds. Add red pepper flakes and rosemary, and stir once. Add tomatoes, along with the juice from one of the cans, and 1 teaspoon of salt. Bring to a boil, then lower heat to medium and simmer, uncovered, stirring occasionally, about 15 to 20 minutes or until sauce begins to thicken.

Place eggplant slices in a single layer on a baking sheet. (You'll need to cook them in several batches.) Cook eggplant slices under the broiler, turning over once, until they are golden brown and tender, about 3 minutes per side. Continue until all eggplant slices have been cooked.

Lower oven heat to 400° F.

In a cheese bowl, stir together ricotta and ½ cup Parmigiano-Reggiano, pepper, and remaining ½ teaspoon of salt. Spray 8-inch x 12-inch baking dish with olive oil spray, and place one-third of the eggplant slices in a layer on the bottom, overlapping slightly. Top with half of the cheese mixture and half of the tomato sauce. Layer half of the remaining eggplant slices over cheese and tomato sauce, then top with the remaining cheese mixture and half of the remaining tomato sauce. Top with the remaining eggplant slices and the rest of the tomato sauce. Sprinkle remaining 2 tablespoons of Parmigiano-Reggiano over the top and bake in preheated oven, uncovered, for about 20 minutes or until bubbly and beginning to brown on top.

Serves 6 to 8.

Broiled Portobello Mushroom "Steaks" with Rosemary-Red Wine Reduction

Meaty Portobello mushrooms are a delicious low-fat, low-calorie alternative to beef. Serve these with a spinach salad and a side of Baked Polenta with Fresh Corn (see recipe, p. 172).

1 tablespoon olive oil
1 medium shallot, finely chopped
1 tablespoon chopped fresh rosemary
½ teaspoon salt
½ teaspoon freshly ground black pepper
2 cups red wine
2 cups vegetable broth
Olive oil spray
4 large portobello mushroom caps, stems removed
2 cloves garlic, minced
2 tablespoons butter

Preheat broiler.

Heat olive oil in a large, heavy skillet over medium-high heat. When oil is hot, add shallot, and cook, stirring until soft, about 3 minutes. Add rosemary, salt, pepper, broth, and wine. Bring to a boil, lower heat, and simmer, uncovered, until reduced by about half, 15 to 20 minutes.

While sauce is cooking, prepare mushrooms. Spray mushroom caps all over with olive oil spray, place cap side down on a baking sheet, sprinkle with minced garlic, and season generously with salt and pepper. Broil under preheated broiler until cooked through, about 8 to 10 minutes.

Just before serving, swirl butter into the hot sauce. Serve mushrooms with sauce drizzled over the top.

Serves 4.

Broiled Tofu and Vegetables
with Peanut Sauce

This quick vegetarian dish is perfect for hurried weekday dinners. Serve with brown rice for a complete meal.

Vegetable oil spray
1 (14- to 16-ounce) package firm tofu, drained and cut into 1-inch thick
    slabs
2 medium zucchini, quartered lengthwise and cut into 3-inch strips
2 medium red bell peppers, seeded and sliced into strips
2 cloves garlic, minced
1 tablespoon minced fresh ginger
½ cup peanut butter (be sure it doesn't have added sugar)
½ cup hot water
2 tablespoons soy sauce
Juice of 1 lime
2 tablespoons fruit sweetener
2 teaspoons sesame oil
1 to 2 teaspoons hot chili oil or chili paste, or to taste
3 green onions, thinly sliced

Preheat broiler. Drain tofu and dry between several layers of paper towels. Spray a baking sheet with vegetable oil spray, and place tofu, zucchini, and bell pepper on the sheet in a single layer. Sprinkle minced garlic and ginger over tofu and vegetables, and spray with vegetable oil spray. Broil in preheated oven for 8 minutes, flip vegetables and tofu over, and continue to cook. Cook another 4 minutes or so until vegetables are soft and beginning to brown. Remove vegetables to a platter, and continue to cook tofu until it is golden brown, about 4 minutes more.

While tofu and vegetables are cooking, whisk together peanut butter and hot water until well combined. Stir in soy sauce, lime juice, fruit sweetener, sesame oil, hot chili oil or chili paste, and green onions.

Serve tofu and peppers on top of steamed brown rice, with peanut sauce drizzled over the top. Place extra peanut sauce in a small bowl to pass at the table.

Serves 4.

24

Side Dishes

Round out your meals with succulent cooked vegetables and hearty whole grains. With these side dish options, you won't miss pasta or bread.

Side Dish Recipes

- Stir Fried Sugar Snap Peas with Garlic
- Roasted Brussels Sprouts with Pine Nuts and Parmesan Cheese
- Roasted Winter Vegetables
  Lemony Green Beans with Toasted Almonds
- Baked Asparagus and Lemon Risotto
  Baked Polenta with Fresh Corn
- Wild Mushroom and Bulgur Stuffing

Stir Fried Sugar Snap Peas with Garlic

A little garlic is all that's needed to dress up crisp, fresh sugar snap peas. Serve these alongside Grilled Chicken Strips with Cilantro Pesto (see recipe, p. 151) on a warm spring or summer evening.

1 tablespoon vegetable oil
3 cloves garlic, peeled and very thinly sliced
1 pound sugar snap peas, trimmed
2 tablespoons water

Heat vegetable oil in a large, heavy skillet over medium-high heat. When oil is hot but not smoking, add the garlic, and cook, stirring about 1 minute. Add peas and cook, stirring about 3 minutes until peas and garlic begin to brown. Add water, cover, and cook until peas are tender, about 5 minutes more.

Roasted Brussels Sprouts with Pine Nuts and Parmesan Cheese

This is an easy and foolproof way to cook Brussels sprouts. Tangy vinegar, crunchy pine nuts, and a dusting of salty Parmesan dress up the sprouts just enough that even skeptics will be sold.

1½ pounds Brussels sprouts, trimmed and halved
1 tablespoon olive oil
1 teaspoon salt
½ teaspoon ground pepper
1/3 cup sherry vinegar
3 tablespoons toasted pine nuts
¼ cup finely grated Parmesan cheese

Preheat oven to 450° F.

In a baking dish, toss together sprouts, oil, salt, and pepper. Spread mixture into a single layer, and roast in oven, stirring once, until sprouts are tender and beginning to brown, about 20 to 25 minutes. Remove from oven and stir in vinegar, scraping up any browned bits from the bottom of the pan. Sprinkle with pine nuts and Parmesan and serve immediately.

Serves 4.

Roasted Winter Vegetables

These are a perfect accompaniment to roasted meats. Any leftovers are great stirred into scrambled eggs or tossed with salad.

2 large orange-fleshed yams, diced
2 large bulbs fennel, cored, thickly sliced
2 medium red onions, thickly sliced
20 large garlic cloves, peeled and left whole
1 tablespoon dried thyme
2 tablespoons olive oil
1½ teaspoons salt
½ teaspoon pepper
½ cup white wine

Preheat oven to 400° F.

In a large baking dish, combine yams, fennel, onions, garlic, and thyme. Toss with olive oil, and sprinkle with salt and pepper. Spread mixture out into an even layer, and roast in a preheated oven, stirring occasionally, until just tender and beginning to brown, about 45 minutes. Stir in wine, and cook another 15 minutes or so, until vegetables are very tender.

Serves 6 to 8.

Lemony Green Beans with Toasted Almonds

Toasted almonds add protein and monounsaturated fat to this light side dish. Serve it alongside a roast chicken with Wild Mushroom and Bulgur Stuffing (see recipe, p. 172) for a simple but elegant family meal.

1 lb. thin green beans such as haricots verts, trimmed
¼ teaspoon salt
¼ teaspoon ground pepper
Juice and zest of ½ lemon
½ tablespoon olive oil
2 tablespoons slivered, toasted almonds

Place beans in a microwave safe bowl and sprinkle with 1 tablespoon of water. Cover bowl with plastic wrap and cook in microwave on high for 3 to 5 minutes, until beans are crisp-tender. Drain beans in colander and return to bowl. Toss with lemon juice, lemon zest, salt, pepper, and olive oil. Serve beans topped with toasted almonds.

Serves 4.

Baked Asparagus and Lemon Risotto

This ingenious preparation takes the stress out of serving risotto for company. The dish can be assembled up to a day ahead of time, then just popped into the oven to bake.

1½ cups aborio or carnaroli rice
1 tablespoon olive oil
1 medium onion, diced
2 cloves garlic, minced
1 pound asparagus, cut into ½-inch pieces
3 eggs, lightly beaten
¼ cup evaporated milk
Juice and finely grated zest of 1 lemon
1½ teaspoons salt
½ teaspoon pepper

1 cup chicken or vegetable broth
Olive oil spray or nonstick cooking spray
6 ounces gruyere cheese, shredded

Preheat oven to 350° F.

Bring 5 cups water to a boil and add rice. Boil rice, stirring occasionally, about 8 minutes, then drain thoroughly.

While rice is boiling, heat olive oil in a heavy skillet over medium-high heat. Add onions and garlic, and cook, stirring about 3 minutes until onions begin to soften. Add asparagus, and cook, stirring about 3 more minutes. Remove from heat and set aside.

In a large bowl, lightly beat eggs, then add evaporated milk, lemon juice and zest, salt, pepper, and broth. Stir in drained rice and asparagus mixture until well combined.

Spray a 9-inch springform pan or cake pan with a removable bottom with olive oil spray or nonstick cooking spray. Wrap a sheet of aluminum foil around the bottom of the pan to catch any drips that might seep through the removable bottom. Pour rice mixture into pan, smooth out into an even layer, and top with shredded cheese. Bake in preheated oven, until cooked through and golden brown on top, about 45 minutes. Remove from oven and let cool slightly before serving.

Serves 4.

Baked Polenta with Fresh Corn

Polenta is a great alternative to pasta when the sauce is the star of the meal. With this simple version, you can pop it in the oven then set about preparing the rest of the meal.

Olive oil spray or vegetable oil spray
1 cup polenta
3½ cups warm water
1 cup fresh corn
1 teaspoon salt
½ cup grated Parmesan cheese

Preheat oven to 350° F.

Spray an 8- x 8-inch baking dish with olive oil spray or nonstick cooking spray and add polenta, water, corn, and salt. Stir to mix. Bake uncovered for about 50 minutes. Stir in Parmesan, and cook another 10 minutes.

Serves 6.

Wild Mushroom and Bulgur Stuffing

This hearty stuffing is a wonderful flour-free alternative to traditional bread stuffing. Serve it with roasted turkey, chicken, or duck. Made with vegetable broth, it's also a festive vegetarian dish.

1½ cups boiling water
4 ounces dried porcini mushrooms
1 tablespoon olive oil
1 medium onion, diced
1 large stalk celery, diced
8 ounces (about 2 cups) cremini or button mushrooms, diced
1 teaspoon dried thyme
1 teaspoon salt
½ teaspoon freshly ground pepper

3 cups chicken or vegetable broth
1¼ cup bulgur

In a bowl, pour boiling water over mushrooms and let soak about 30 minutes. Remove mushrooms from water, reserving soaking liquid, and chop coarsely.

In a large, heavy skillet heat olive oil over medium-high heat. When oil is hot but not smoking, add onion and celery, and cook, stirring until softened, about 5 minutes. Add chopped dried mushrooms along with fresh mushrooms to the pan, and continue to cook, stirring until the fresh mushrooms give up their liquid and it begins to evaporate. Stir in thyme, salt, and pepper. Add the soaking liquid from the dried mushrooms to the pan, being careful to leave any sandy grit behind, along with the broth. Bring to a boil, and stir in bulgur. Return to a boil, then lower heat to medium, and simmer uncovered about 6 to 8 minutes.

To cook the stuffing outside of the poultry (recommended): Spread stuffing in a shallow baking dish and cook, covered, in a preheated 400° oven for 35 to 40 minutes.

To cook stuffing inside poultry: Just before cooking, loosely fill the bird's body cavity with stuffing. Be sure to cook until the meat is completely cooked. (It should reach 180° F on a meat thermometer.) The stuffing should reach a temperature of 160° F.

Serves 4 to 6.

Desserts

Most of us have a sweet tooth, and the truth of the matter is that denying ourselves dessert only sets us up for unmitigated bingeing. These sweet treats will keep you satisfied without knocking you off the no flour, no sugar wagon.

Dessert Recipes

- Cinnamon-Poached Pears
- Banana Nut "Ice Cream"
- Lemon Panna Cotta with Raspberry Coulis
- Peach and Blueberry Crisp
- Strawberry Crepes with Dark Chocolate Sauce
- Dark Chocolate Sauce

Cinnamon-Poached Pears

The apple juice and wine cook down to a rich, caramel-like syrup. On their own, these pears are a sweet, low-calorie way to end a meal. For a special treat, try them drizzled with Dark Chocolate Sauce (see recipe, p. 178) or topped with a scoop of no-sugar-added vanilla ice cream or frozen yogurt.

    1 cup apple juice
    1 cup white wine
    ¼ cup fruit sweetener
    1 cinnamon stick
    4 ripe pears, peeled, halved, and cored

In a large, heavy saucepan, combine apple juice, wine, fruit sweetener, and cinnamon stick, and bring to a boil over medium-high heat. Simmer, stirring frequently, until sauce begins to thicken, about 5 minutes. Add pears to saucepan, and spoon some of the sauce over them. Cover pan, reduce heat to medium-low, and simmer until pears are tender, about 8 minutes.

Serves 4.

Banana Nut "Ice Cream"

This guilt-free frozen dessert is sure to satisfy your sweet tooth. For a special treat, serve it drizzled with Dark Chocolate Sauce (see recipe, p. 178). You may need to remove it from the freezer and let it soften a few minutes before serving.

    4 medium, very ripe bananas
    2 tablespoons fruit sweetener
    2 tablespoons water
    2 tablespoons chopped toasted walnuts

Place bananas, fruit sweetener, and water in a blender or food processor and process until mostly smooth. Stir in walnut pieces and pour mixture into a medium bowl or 4 individual serving dishes. Cover with plastic wrap and freeze, stirring every 30 minutes, for 2 hours. Serve immediately—or keep frozen for several weeks.

Serves 4.

Lemon Panna Cotta
with Raspberry Coulis

This light Italian-style milk pudding is a great way to get some of your daily calcium. The gorgeous jewel-colored raspberry sauce is also delicious drizzled over sugar-free vanilla ice cream or stirred into nonfat plain yogurt.

For Panna Cotta:
1 envelope powdered gelatin
1½ tablespoons water
2 cups low-fat milk (1%)
2 teaspoons vanilla extract
Finely grated zest of 1 lemon
¼ cup fruit sweetener

For Raspberry Coulis:
1 12-ounce bag frozen, unsweetened raspberries, thawed
½ cup fruit sweetener
½ cup hot water, or more if needed to achieve desired consistency

Place the gelatin and 1½ tablespoons water in a saucepan over low heat and stir until gelatin has dissolved. Add milk, vanilla extract, lemon zest, and ¼ cup fruit sweetener. Cook over medium-low heat for about 5 minutes until mixture is hot to the touch. Pour the mixture into 6 custard cups, ½-cup ramekins, or even small coffee cups, and refrigerate for at least 4 hours or as long as overnight.

Place raspberries, fruit sweetener, and water in food processor or blender and puree until smooth. Strain the mixture through a fine-mesh sieve to remove the seeds. Coulis can be served immediately or refrigerated up to one week. Bring to room temperature before serving.

To serve, unmold custards onto dessert plates, drizzle some of the coulis over and around the custard, and, if desired, garnish with a fresh mint sprig.

Serves 6.

Peach and Blueberry Crisp

Peaches and blueberries celebrate the height of summer, but this simple dessert can be easily adapted for whatever fruit you have available—nectarines, apricots, apples, pears, etc.

3 tablespoons butter
1 cup almond meal
3 tablespoons fruit sweetener

4 medium, ripe peaches, peeled, pitted, and thinly sliced
1 cup fresh, ripe blueberries

Preheat oven to 400° F.

In a food processor, combine butter and almond meal until butter is fully incorporated. Add fruit sweetener and process until well combined.

Mix sliced peaches and blueberries together and place in 9-inch pie dish. Top with almond meal mixture, dolloping it around and evenly distributing it over the fruit. Bake in preheated oven for 8 to 10 minutes, until topping is lightly browned and crisp.

Serves 4.

Strawberry Crepes
with Dark Chocolate Sauce

You could substitute any ripe fresh fruit, like bananas or pears, but strawberries make for an especially pretty dish.

Basic Crepes (see recipe, p. 111)
1 pint fresh, ripe strawberries, stemmed and sliced
Dark Chocolate Sauce (recipe below)

Prepare Dark Chocolate Sauce and Basic Crepes according to recipes. Divide strawberries evenly among the crepes, arranging them down the middle of the crepes, and roll the crepes up around them. Drizzle about 2 tablespoons of chocolate sauce decoratively over each rolled-up crepe. Serve immediately.

Serves 6.

Dark Chocolate Sauce

This rich sauce is delicious drizzled over Strawberry Crepes (recipe above), Cinnamon Poached Pears (see recipe, p. 175), or simply used as a dip for fresh fruit. Using low-fat evaporated milk and fruit sweetener significantly cuts calories while still delivering creamy sweetness. Remember, though, that baking chocolate is high in fat, which means it still packs a fairly hefty calorie punch. Use this sauce sparingly.

½ cup evaporated milk
½ cup fruit sweetener
1 teaspoon vanilla extract
3 ounces unsweetened baking chocolate, roughly chopped

Place chocolate in a non-reactive bowl. Place milk and fruit sweetener in a small saucepan over medium-high heat and heat until hot to the touch but not boiling. Pour hot milk over chocolate in bowl, add vanilla extract, and let sit a few minutes until chocolate has softened. Stir until chocolate has melted completely. Serve sauce immediately, or cover and refrigerate up to one week. To serve, heat in microwave just until hot and liquid.

Index

A

acorn squash 52, 87
Adderal 67
addiction 67
aerobics 46
agave cactus nectar 91
alcohol 9, 73, 79, 88
algae 71
all-purpose flour 16
allergies 50
almonds 53, 55, 87, 97, 103
amazake 92
American Heart Association 36, 61, 64
amino acid 67
anemia 69
angustofolia 70
animal fat 62
ankle swelling 85
antioxidants 11, 70, 74
anxiety 44, 67, 70
appetite suppressants 67
appetizers 133, 138
apple cider vinegar 69
apple juice 91
apples 20, 52, 55, 87, 90, 100, 102, 156, 177
apricots 20, 52, 55, 87, 90, 103, 177
arrowroot powder 87
arteries 59, 61, 63, 76
arthritis 45, 73
artichokes 19
artificial sweeteners 5, 51
Asian Americans 58
Asian seasonings 118
asparagus 19, 52, 101
aspartame 93, 95
aspartic acid 93
asphyxiation 70
atherosclerosis 59, 60
Atkins diet 35, 73, 76
avocados 11, 19, 52, 72, 87

B

backpacking 45
bacon 62
bagels 86
Baked Asparagus and Lemon Risotto 167, 170
Baked Eggs with Canadian Bacon, Tomatoes and Feta 100, 107, 115
Baked Halibut with Fennel, Sun Dried Tomatoes, and Olives 140, 141
Baked Polenta with Fresh Corn 100, 152, 164, 167
Baked Tortilla Chips 102, 103, 133, 135, 136
ballroom dance 45
balsamic vinaigrette 100, 101, 103
balsamic vinegar 53
Banana Nut "Ice Cream" 174, 175
bananas 20, 53, 72, 87, 100-03, 109, 110

barley 5, 9, 14, 15, 16, 19, 51, 87, 96
barley flour 17
barley, sprouted 97
Basic Crepes 101, 103, 107, 111
basketball 46
beans 9, 12, 19, 37, 72, 87, 96
beef 52, 62, 88
beef stroganoff 77
beet sugar 5, 13, 17, 34
bell peppers 52, 55, 87, 101, 130, 138
bernaise sauce 63
berries 53, 87, 90
bike 64
bike, stationary 47
biking 46, 48
birthdays 62, 79
Black Bean Salad 116, 123
black people 58
blackberries 53
bloating 69, 95
blood cholesterol 44
blood cholesterol level 62
blood clots 67
blood fat levels 35
blood glucose levels 57
blood pressure 11, 60
blood sugar 15, 35, 57, 58, 69, 85
blueberries 20, 53, 74
body fat 68, 69, 71
Body Mass Index (BMI) 27
bones 11, 75
bones, brittle 73
bowel function 37
Brazil 91
breads 16, 38, 50, 78, 86, 167
breakfast 107
broccoli 19, 52, 87, 103, 112
Broiled Portobello Mushroom "Steaks" with Rosemary-Red Wine Reduction 101, 140, 164
Broiled Tofu and Vegetables with Peanut Sauce 140, 165
brown rice 5, 15, 96
brown rice flour 17
brown rice syrup 17, 92
brown sugar 17
brunch 113, 114
Brussels sprouts 52, 87
buckthorn 70
buckwheat 16
bulgur 19, 51, 87, 97
burgers 78
butter 53, 61, 62, 97
butternut 87
butternut squash 52

C

cabbage 52, 87
caffeine 70

cake flour 17
cakes 14, 86
calcium 68, 73, 75
calisthenics 49
cancer 9, 75
cancer, colon 73
candy 14, 53, 86, 94
cane sugar 5, 13, 17, 34, 89, 90
canola oil 11, 19, 88
cantaloupe 20, 53, 55, 100
carbo-phobia 73
carbohydrates 9, 14, 19, 36, 56, 92, 94, 96, 97, 107
carbohydrates, complex 14, 57
cardiovascular disease 61, 98
cardiovascular risk 11
carrots 19, 55, 87, 97, 100, 138
cascara 70
cashews 87
cassia angustofolia 70
cauliflower 19, 52, 87, 103
celery 19, 52, 55, 87, 101, 102, 138
cereals 16, 38, 51
chard 87
cheese 51, 61, 62, 88, 97, 100, 101, 102, 103, 111
cherries 20, 53, 55, 87, 90
chewing gum 5
chicken 19, 88, 100, 101, 102, 122, 123, 126, 128, 161
Chicken Breasts in Rosemary-Dijon Sauce 140, 147
chicken noodle soup 77
Chile-Lime Roasted Chickpeas and Pistachios 101, 102, 133, 134
chili dipping sauce 78
Chilled Cucumber Soup with Avocado and Mint 116, 117
Chinese restaurants 78
Chipotle Tomato and Corn Bisque 103, 116, 120
chitosan 69
choking 70
cholesterol 6, 9, 15, 35, 36, 44, 56, 58, 59, 60, 61, 63, 69, 70, 73, 75
chow mein 77
chromium picolinate 69
chromium supplements 69
cigarettes 67
Cinnamon Poached Pears 174, 175, 178
citrus fruits 90
clams 52
coach 46
Cobb Salad Wrap 102, 116, 129
Coconut-Pecan Granola 100, 102, 107, 108
cod 52
coffee 90, 93
coffee, decaffeinated 78
colon cancer 44

complex sugars 14
concentrated sugar 5
congestive heart failure 63
constipation 71, 73
cookies 14, 16, 50, 86, 94
corn 5, 14, 19, 78, 87, 96
corn bran 16
corn chips 64
corn flour 5, 16, 17, 78, 96
corn meal 16, 87, 96
corn oil margarine 62
corn oils 11
corn syrup 5, 13, 17, 34, 50, 89, 90, 96
corn tortillas 51, 96
cornmeal mush 97
coronary heart disease 6, 59, 63
crab 52, 88
crab cakes 97
crackers 16, 86
cream cheese 62
Crohn's disease 73
croissants 86
cross-country skiing 48
croutons 77
cucumber 19, 101
Curried Lentils with Butternut Squash 102, 140, 160
Curry Yogurt Chicken 101, 140, 149

D
dairy products 9, 12, 93
dancing 46
Dark Chocolate Sauce 174, 175
deficiencies 71
depression 44
dessert 78, 174
dextrose 92
diabetes 6, 9, 37, 44, 56, 57, 58, 67, 68, 75
diabetics 58, 59
diarrhea 69, 95
diastolic pressure 63
Diet Coke 91
diet goals 54
diet plan 26, 50, 82
dietary fat 73
dietary guidelines 9
Dietary Guidelines for Americans 2005 48
dietary supplement 91
digestive disorder 37
digestive process 15
digestive system 68, 70
dinner, light 131
diuretics 68
diverticulitis 73
DNA damage 69
donuts 86
dried fruit 108
dumplings 78

E

eating patterns 30, 31, 32, 33
Edamame 53
egg rolls 78
egg salad 63
egg substitute 51
egg yolks 63, 71
eggplant 19, 52
Eggplant and Tomato Spread 100, 121, 133, 137
Eggplant "Lasagne" 140
eggs 51, 61, 63, 72, 88, 101, 103
empty calories 6, 13, 16-19, 75, 88, 94
endive 52, 55, 87, 137, 138
English peas 87
entrees 140
ephedrine 69
Equal 93
esophagus 70
evaporated cane juice 17
exercise 44, 46, 47, 48, 49, 54, 58, 60, 61, 64, 72, 74, 75, 79, 85

F

fad diets 4, 6, 9, 81
fast food 42, 50, 63, 66
fatigue 57
fats 9, 19, 118, 127, 136, 147
FDA 36, 37, 71, 72, 94
Feta Cheese Omelet with Zucchini, Peas, and Mint 107, 113
fiber 11, 13, 15, 16, 37, 62, 69, 70, 73, 90, 110, 136, 150
fiber supplements 70
figs 52, 87, 90
fish 19, 52, 61, 66, 71, 72, 78, 88, 98, 99, 122, 126
flour, cake 86
flour, all-purpose 86
flour, brown rice 86
flour, corn 86
flour, pastry 16, 86
flour, rice 86
flour, rye 17, 86
flour, unbleached 17, 86
flour, wheat 5, 16
flour, whole wheat 16, 86
food groups 6
food journal 30, 31, 32
food sensitivities 50
fried foods 62
Frittata with Tender Greens and Fontina Cheese 102, 107, 114
fructose 5, 17, 53, 89, 90
fruit 5, 19, 55, 66, 77, 89, 98, 110
fruit crisp 108
fruit juices 91
fruit pie 78
fruit preserves 53, 87, 90
Fruit Sweet 91
fruit sweeteners 51, 88, 91
fruits 6, 9, 11, 13, 14, 15, 20, 37, 55, 60, 62, 70, 73, 75, 87, 93, 95, 96
fruits, dried 87, 90
Fusion Gazpacho with Seafood 102, 103, 116, 118

G

garbanzo beans 52
gardening 46
gas 69
gastrointestinal distress 72
Glucommannan (konjac) 70
glucose 5, 13, 14, 15, 17, 34, 89
goal weight 26, 99
golf 46
gout 73
grains 9, 71, 93
grape leaves 121
grapefruit-diet pills 70
grapes 53, 55, 87, 90
Greek Salad 100, 103, 116, 121, 122
green beans 52, 87, 149
Green Chile and Cheese Quesadillas 102, 116, 130
green salad 77, 100, 101, 103
green tea 70
greens, leafy 19, 52
Grilled Chicken Strips with Cilantro-Lime Pesto 140, 151, 168
growth hormone releasers 70
guar gum 70
guarana 69

H

ham 62, 101, 103, 111
hamburger 62
hand weights 47
hardening of the arteries 59
hazelnuts 97
HDL (the "good" cholesterol) 11, 36, 60, 61
headaches 69
health food stores 92
heart attack 36, 60, 61, 63
heart disease 9, 36, 44, 59, 61, 68, 73, 74, 75
heartbeat, irregular 67
Hearty Four-Grain Cereal 101, 102, 107, 109
hemorrhoids 73
herbal cocktails 69
herbs 52, 55, 69
heroin 67
high blood pressure 37, 44, 58, 60, 63, 85
high-density lipoprotein. See HDL
hiking 45, 46, 64
hip hop dance 45
Hispanics 58
hockey 45
hoisin sauce 78, 86

holidays 62, 63, 79
hollandaise sauce 63
honey 5, 13, 17, 34, 50, 90, 91, 92
honeydew melon 20, 53, 55
hors d'ouevre 138
hot pepper sauce 53
hotdogs 62
human growth hormone (HGH) 70
hummus 53, 101, 138
hunger 57, 69
hydrogenated oil 11
hypertension 6, 37, 44, 56, 60, 63, 64, 70, 73

I
ice cream 53, 62, 86, 88, 94, 175
imbalances 71, 75
immune system 66
insomnia 67, 70
insulin 11, 57, 58, 59
internal organs 11
iodine 71
irritable bowel syndrome 73
Italian restaurants 78, 97

J
jams 50, 53, 86
Japan 91
Japanese restaurants 78
Jello 53
jelly 86
jitteriness 67
jogging 46
Johns Hopkins University 92
junk food 79, 133

K
kale 52, 87
kelp 71
kidney beans 52
kidney damage 97
kidney disease 37
kidney stones 73
kola nut, 69
konjac 70

L
lactitol 94
lactose 89
Laughing Cow Light Cheese 102
laxatives 68
LDL (the "bad" cholesterol) 11, 36, 61, 62
lecithin 71
legumes 9, 13, 14, 15, 19, 71, 73, 75, 87
lemon juice 55
Lemon Panna Cotta with Raspberry Coulis
    174, 176
lemon sauce 78
Lemony Green Beans with Toasted Almonds
    167, 170

lentils 52
lettuce 52, 78, 87
lima beans 97
line dancing 45
lipotropic "fat burners" 71
liquid egg substitute 88
liquid-diet drink 72
liver 61, 73
liver damage 67, 97
locust plant 70
London Broil 88
Louisiana 146
low-density lipoprotein. See LDL
low-fat dairy products 19
low-fat milk 9, 14, 20
lunch 116, 117, 121, 131
lunch meats 52, 62

M
ma huang 69
macaroni and cheese 62
mackerel 88
macronutrients 9, 12, 19
magnesium 68
malted barley flour 16
maltitol 94
mangoes 55, 87
maple syrup 5, 13, 17, 34, 50, 90, 92
margarine 62
mayonnaise 53, 63
meal plan 50, 55, 76
meal-replacement liquids 71
meat 12, 19, 20, 61, 63, 66, 72, 78, 88, 93, 98
Meatballs in Tomato Sauce 100, 140, 152
meatloaf 97
Mediterranean-style diet 11
melons 53, 87, 90, 102
memory loss 69
metabolism 70, 74, 93
methamphetamines 67
Mexican restaurants 78
Middle Eastern spices 121
milk 61, 62, 88, 100, 101, 102, 103, 108
milk products 14
milk, skim 51
milk sugar (lactose) 89
minerals 12, 13, 16
mint 52
mirin 154
miso soup 53
molasses 5, 17, 34, 50, 90, 92
monounsaturated fats 11, 134
Moroccan Chicken Stew with Butternut
    Squash and Quinoa 103, 140, 150
mountain biking 45
mozzarella cheese 101, 102
muscle mass 69
muscle tissue 74
muscles 11, 71

Mushroom Soup with Barley 100, 116, 119
mushrooms 52, 112
Mushrooms Stuffed with Corn and Goat
    Cheese 103, 133, 138
mussels 52, 88
mustard 53
MyPyramid 9

N
National Diabetes Information Clearinghouse
    57
Native Americans 58
"natural" weight loss aids 69
nectarines 20, 52, 55, 87, 90, 177
nerve damage 72
nervousness 67, 69, 70
nicotine 67
nitrogen 74
nonfat milk 9, 14, 20
noodles 53, 77
numbness 72
nut butters 53, 87
nut meal 97
Nutrasweet 88, 93
nutrient-dense foods 12, 16, 18, 19, 75, 89
nutrients 9, 67, 68, 71, 74, 75, 90, 150
nutrition 75
nutrition labels 34, 36
nuts 11, 12, 19, 20, 53, 55, 72, 87

O
OA. See Overeaters Anonymous
oat bran 16
Oatmeal Pancakes 107, 110
oats 9, 14, 15, 16, 19, 72, 87, 96
obesity 11, 24, 27, 57
obstruction 70
olive oil 11, 19, 53, 62, 88
Omelet Muffins 103, 107, 112
onions 52, 101
optimal weight 26, 30, 40
orange sauce 78
oranges 20, 53
oregano 52
osteoporosis 73
Overeaters Anonymous 43
oysters 88

P
Pacific Islanders 58
Pad Thai 78
palpitations 70
Pan Roasted Chicken with Bacon, Olives, and
    Prunes 140, 148
pancreas 57, 58
papayas 55, 87
Paraguay 91
partially hydrogenated oil 11
pasilla chiles 130

pasta 16, 50, 56, 77, 82, 86, 97, 99, 167
pastries 50
Peach and Blueberry Crisp 174, 177
peaches 20, 52, 55, 87, 90, 100, 102, 108,
    110, 111
peanut butter 50, 53, 87, 100, 102
peanut sauce 78
peanuts 71
pears 20, 55, 87, 90, 177
peas 19, 87, 96, 97
pecans 87
pectin 69
pepperoni 62
peppers 112
phenylalanine 67, 93
phenylpropanolamine (PPA) 67, 70
phytochemicals 11, 74
pickle relish 53
pickles, dill 53
pineapple 87, 100
pistachios 53, 55, 87
pituitary gland 70
pizza 62, 66, 78
plaque 60, 61
plum sauce 78
plums 20, 55, 90
poblano or pasilla chiles 130
polenta 51, 87, 97
polyphenols 70
polyunsaturated 11
pork chops 88
pork tenderloin 52, 88
Pork Tenderloin Roasted with Fennel, Apples,
    Potatoes and Onions 103, 140, 156
portion control 39, 40
pot pie 78
pot stickers 78
potassium 68, 70
potato chips 64
potatoes 5, 56, 72, 79, 87, 96, 97, 101
poultry 12, 20, 52, 61, 78, 88, 98
processed foods 6
protein 9, 12, 19, 36, 66, 71, 73, 107, 118,
    134, 136, 150
pudding 50, 53, 88
pumpkin 52, 87
pumpkin seeds 87
pyridoxine 72

Q
quiche 78
quinoa 14, 19, 51, 87, 97, 100, 101, 103, 140,
    150

R
Radicchio Salad with Pears, Blue Cheese, and
    Toast 100, 116, 126
radishes 52, 55, 87
raisins 108, 121

raspberries 20, 53
resistance exercises 49
respiratory disorder 67
rice 9, 14, 16, 51, 56, 79, 87, 92, 96, 102, 103
rice, brown 19, 77, 100, 101, 102, 145, 149, 154, 165
rice flour 5, 16, 17, 78
Rice Krispies 94
rice noodle dishes 78
risotto 78, 87, 97
Ritalin 67
Roasted Brussels Sprouts with Pine Nuts and Parmesan Cheese 102, 167, 168
Roasted Garlic Salmon 100, 140, 142
Roasted Winter Vegetables 102, 167, 169
rock climbing 45
root vegetables 19
running 45, 46
rye 16
rye, sprouted 97

S
saccharin 92
safflower oil 11, 53, 88
salad dressing 53, 86, 94
salads 98
salmon 52, 88
salsa 53, 124
sandwiches 78, 82, 97, 116
saturated fats 9, 11, 12, 35, 36, 60, 61, 73, 75
sausage 62
scallops 52, 88
seafood 11, 12, 20, 88
Seared Ahi Tuna with Wasabi Sauce 103, 140, 144
Seared Pork Chops with Cherry-Balsamic Reduction 101, 140, 157
Seared Salmon Fillets with Sorrel-Tomato Compote 101, 140, 143
seaweed 71
seeds 12, 19, 20, 72, 87
self-esteem 85
senna 70
sesame seeds 87
shellfish 52, 69, 88
Shepherd's Pie 140, 158
sherbet 62
shopping list 51
shrimp 52, 88, 123, 151
side dishes 167
skating 48
skim milk 53
skin 11
sleeplessness 67, 69, 72
snacking 54, 55, 133, 134
snow peas 87
soba noodle soup 78
soccer 45
sodas 86

sodas, diet 88
sodium 37, 60, 64
softball 45
sorbet 62
sorbitol 94
Sores 58
soups 53
sour cream 53
soy 74
soy beans 53
soy grits 16
soy nuts 20, 53, 87
soy products 20
soy sauce 53, 91
soy-based sausage 52
soybeans 71
speed 67
Spiced Edamame 100, 101, 133, 134
Spiced Pumpkin Dip 101, 103, 133, 138
spinach 52, 87
spinach salad 142, 164
Spinach Salad with Tomato Vinaigrette 100, 116, 127
spirulina 71
Splenda 5, 78, 88, 90, 93
spring rolls 78
squash 19, 52, 87
St. John's Wort 72
starch blockers 71
stevia 51, 88, 91
Stir Fried Sugar Snap Peas with Garlic 101, 167, 168
Stir-Fried Beef with Sugar Snap Peas 102, 140, 154
strawberries 20, 53, 55, 100, 103, 108, 110
Strawberry Crepes with Dark Chocolate Sauce 174, 178
stress 44, 64
stretching 45, 47, 49
stroke 36, 37, 44, 61, 63, 75
substance abuse 68
sucralose 93, 95
sucrose 5, 17, 34, 89, 90, 95
sugar 50
sugar alcohol 95
sugar alcohols 94
sugar, raw 17
sugar, refined 5
sugar snap peas 87
sugar-free soda 5
sugars, simple 13
summer rolls 78
Summer Salsa 102, 133, 135, 136
sunflower oil 53, 88
sunflower seeds 87
sweet chili dipping sauce 78
Sweet 'N Low 92
sweet potatoes 87
sweet tooth 89, 174

sweeteners 17, 53, 78, 88, 90, 91
sweeteners, natural 89, 92
sweeteners, no-calorie 75
swimming 46, 48
systolic pressure 63

T

Taco Salad with Spiced Prawns 101, 116, 124, 135
tacos 135
tahini (sesame paste) 87
Take Off Pounds Sensibly. See TOPS
tart 78
tea 78, 91
tea, diet 69
tennis 5
tension 64
tequila 91
teriyaki sauce 78, 86
Thai restaurant 78
Thai-Style Coleslaw 116, 128
Thai-Style Shrimp in Coconut Milk 140, 145
thirst 57
throat 70
thyroid disorders 67
thyroid gland 71
tiredness 72
tofu 19, 20, 52, 123, 151
tofu hot dogs 52
tomatillo, green 124
tomatoes 19, 52, 87, 100, 101
TOPS 43
tortilla chips 78, 86, 97, 124
trainer 46
trans fats 9, 35, 36, 61
treadmill 5, 45, 47
triglycerides 69, 70
trout, 52
tuna 52, 100, 101
turkey 52, 88, 102
Turkey Sausage, Shrimp, and Brown Rice Jambalaya 140, 146
Two-Bean Salad 116, 121

U

U.S. Food and Drug Administration 37
udon 78
United States Department of Agriculture (USDA) 8, 9, 40
unsaturated fats 11, 107
uric acid 73
urination, increased 57
USDA Dietary Guidelines for Americans 46

V

vacations 79
vegetable oil 11
vegetables 6, 9, 11, 13, 14, 15, 19, 37, 54, 55, 60, 62, 66, 70, 73, 75, 77, 87, 90, 95, 96, 97,
100, 101, 103, 156, 167
veggie pepperoni 52
Vietnamese Shrimp Wraps 101, 116, 131
vinaigrette dressing 100
vision, blurred 58
vitamin A 75
Vitamin B$_6$ 72
vitamin D 75
vitamins 12, 13, 16, 66, 69, 90
vitamins A, D, E, and K 11

W

walking 5, 45, 46, 48, 64
walnuts 87
water weight 25, 68, 74
watermelon 53
Wax Orchard brand 91
weddings 79
weigh-in, weekly 82
weight lifting 45
weight loss 25, 26, 29, 35, 40, 42, 44, 57, 58, 68, 69, 70, 71, 72, 73, 79, 81, 82
weight loss organizations 43
wheat 9, 14, 15
wheat berries 5
wheat berries, sprouted 97
wheat bran 16
"wheat breads" 16
wheat germ 71
wheat grain 15
White Bean Stew 140, 161
whole grain cereal 100, 103
whole grains 5, 6, 9, 11, 13, 14, 15, 16, 19, 37, 60, 62, 73, 75, 167
whole grains, sprouted 97
whole wheat bread 96
whole wheat pasta 96
whole-grain hot cereal 94
whole-milk products 63
Wild Mushroom and Bulgur Stuffing 102, 167, 172
wine, red 74, 88
wine, white 154
wurst 62

Y

yams 19, 87, 101
yard work 46
yeast 71
"yo-yo" effect 72
yoga 45
yogurt 51, 55, 88, 100, 108, 110, 111
yogurt, frozen 53, 62, 175

Z

Zesty Black Bean Dip 102, 103, 133, 135, 136
zinc 68, 75
zucchini 87, 101

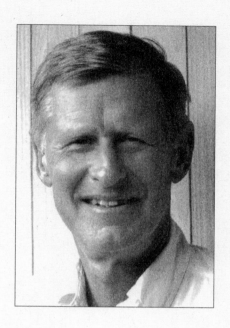

About the Author

Peter H. Gott, MD, is America's most popular medical columnist. His column appears in more than 350 newspapers worldwide. Dr. Gott has had a solo family/general practice in rural Connecticut since 1966 and recently retired as the medical director of the Hotchkiss School, a coed preparatory boarding school in his community.

Dr. Gott has been published in the *New England Journal of Medicine, USA Today, Saturday Review, Working Mother, Lancet, Patient Care,* and a host of other periodicals. His other books include *No House Calls: Irreverent Notes on the Practice of Medicine, Summer Windows of 'Sconset, and Live Longer, Live Better: Taking Care of Your Health.*